May you always feel blessed!
Faith Anderson

Help Me, Lord!
I'm Too Stressed to Feel Blessed

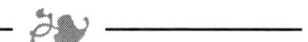

Faith Anderson

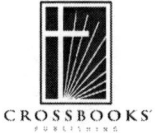

CrossBooks™
A Division of LifeWay
1663 Liberty Drive
Bloomington, IN 47403
www.crossbooks.com
Phone: 1-866-879-0502

©2011 Faith Anderson. All rights reserved.

No part of this book may be reproduced, stored in a retrieval system, or transmitted by any means without the written permission of the author.

First published by CrossBooks 06/27/2011

ISBN: 978-1-4627-0518-4 (sc)
ISBN: 978-1-4627-0519-1 (hc)

Library of Congress Control Number: 2011933029

Scripture taken from The Living Bible The Way

Printed in the United States of America

This book is printed on acid-free paper.

Any people depicted in stock imagery provided by Thinkstock are models, and such images are being used for illustrative purposes only.

Certain stock imagery © Thinkstock.

Because of the dynamic nature of the Internet, any web addresses or links contained in this book may have changed since publication and may no longer be valid. The views expressed in this work are solely those of the author and do not necessarily reflect the views of the publisher, and the publisher hereby disclaims any responsibility for them.

To God

I was not raised in a godly home. My first introduction to God was the film reels that were played for the kids at the county fair. The person running the tape would encourage the little children to come into the tent and watch a short film about Jesus. Later, there was a local church with a bus ministry, and they stopped at our house to say that if any member of our family wanted to go to church, they would take us. My younger sister, Karen and I ventured to church on our own in this way, and there we found Jesus. I became saved around the age of 10. As the country singer, Rascal Flatts would say, "God bless the broken road that led me straight to you (Jesus)." I wish I could say that I had always remained faithful to God since my salvation, but I did not. I took many detours, and only by God's grace have I arrived at where I am now.

I met my husband at age 16. Bob and I have been married for 25 years, and live in Greencastle, Pa. God knew what I needed in my life and so he placed me in this marriage, not only with a loving husband, but with a godly, Christian mother in law, who has been a wonderful example for me to follow. My husband Bob and I have two daughters, and five grandchildren. I graduated from nursing school in 1984 as a Licensed Practical Nurse, and continue to work full time in a busy physician's office. I also recently received my certificate as a basic Lay Speaker for my church. I am proud to say that I am a cancer survivor. I was diagnosed with Acute Myeloid Leukemia (AML) in 2001, and after six courses of chemotherapy, I have been cancer free for 10 years.

This book was written as a result of my plea with God, to show me areas in my life where I needed to improve. I had become so focused on the world around me, and the stress of everyday life, that I was no longer able to have a close relationship with God. I felt completely overwhelmed on a daily basis, trying to get everything done at home, at work, and with my family. God showed me that these areas are common to many of today's women. He, then led me through biblical scriptures to find the answers I needed to get my life back in order, and he showed me how these scriptures pertain to the current times that we are living in. My hope is that these short stories will enable you to look at your life differently, and that you will be able to feel more relaxed, and blessed as a result of them.

May God Bless You,

Faith

Contents

1. Children 1
2. Church 3
3. Fear 6
4. Thoughts 9
5. Desires 12
6. Priorities 15
7. Judging 18
8. Laughter 20
9. Love 23
10. Marriage 26
11. Neighbors 29
12. Guidance 32
13. Parents 35
14. Problems 38
15. Purpose 41
16. Respect 43
17. Protection 46
18. Satisfaction 49
19. Size 52
20. Grace 55
21. Words 58
22. Stumbling Block 61
23. Sickness 64
24. Temptations 67
25. Tithes 70
26. Waiting 73
27. Whispers 77
28. Willing Hands 80
29. Worry 83
30. Joy 86

Bob,

Thank you for all of your love and patience.

Glenda, Gloria, Charlie, Jean, Kristen, Lewis, Tonia, Brandi,

Thank you for all of your encouragement and support.

1.
Children

In 1980, there was a song released by Dr. Hook called "Girls Can Get It." The lyrics said that all a girl had to do was snap her fingers and she could make a boy run to her at the speed of light. In a lot of ways, this is still true today. Girls can get a lot of attention, whether they intend to or not.

God blessed me with two daughters, and two beautiful granddaughters. I also have three young grandsons. I have watched as one daughter tries to train her three sons to respect women, and the other daughter tries to train her two daughters to respect themselves. It's difficult to bring up a child that God has entrusted to you in this world and try to do it right. There are too many negative influences on our children, everything, from music videos, You-Tube, and even fashion trends.

Do we as parents really need our young girls wearing "skinny jeans" and crop tops that show off their belly button rings? Young kids are also being left home alone after school with unsupervised access to the Internet, and some of the shows on TV that are not fit for our kids to watch.

We have to be diligent with our children and our grandchildren. They can think of things that we would never dream of, and they know a lot of things that we don't understand. If you don't believe me, just watch our kids or grand-kids with their IPods and video games. We need to monitor what they listen to and what games they play.

One Sunday morning, I came out of the bathroom after getting ready for church, to find my nine year old granddaughter watching an MTV music video of the song "F -You." Really! What happened to the sweet little girl watching cartoons when I went into the bathroom! Needless to say, she tried to tell me she was allowed to watch this, which I knew was not true. So after she and I talked, we (her parents, her grandfather, and I) made a point of sitting down with her to discuss this. You see, this way we stay united. We need these children to know that if it's wrong at home, it's also wrong everywhere else, whether it is at grandma's house, school, or a friends' house.

Family life runs so much smoother if children are taught boundaries, and these limits are reinforced. We are the grownups. I know it will make for a much calmer atmosphere at home if the kids are allowed to do as they please; but in the long run they will become much better adults if they know there are limits, and that certain actions result in definite consequences.

We need to not only monitor the music that our children listen to, and the games they play, but also to their interactions with each other. We can't allow our sons to grow up bullying other children. We need to teach them respect for each other, and for other people's property.

We need to teach our young girls how to dress in a modest fashion, so as not to attract the attention of males, young and old alike. The male attention might be a self-esteem boost for the girls, knowing that they were able to turn heads, but these girls aren't physically or emotionally ready to handle the sexual consequences that could come from it. Not only the emotional upheaval it can bring, but also the possible sexually transmitted diseases, or teen pregnancy. I have seen the fashion trends for our younger generation. It's hard for girls to put together a decent outfit, and still look cute, and have everything covered at the same time.

We have to remember that God entrusted this child to us for their upbringing, and this is quite possibly the most important job we will ever have. We have to remain focused on their wellbeing, and set boundaries, so that they grow into godly men and women.

❧ Proverbs 22:6

"Train up a child in the way he should go; and
when he is old, he will not depart from it."

2.
Church

Many people do not go to church. They say they don't need it, so why go. They say that the only people who go to church are hypocrites. That some of the people in church have no right to be there because of the things they've done in the past. We've all heard the excuses, and the list of all the wrongs that "Christians" do.

What these people don't realize is that church is not for the perfect people. Church is for the broken, damaged, hurting people. If church were only for the "perfect" people, there would be nobody there on Sunday mornings, probably not even the preacher!

Romans 3:23 "For everyone has sinned and have fallen short of the Glory of God." These are the people Jesus came to save. Where else are they to go, but to the only one who can help them?

A lot of people mistakenly feel they don't need to go to church. They believe in Jesus, and they believe they are a good person, so they will go to heaven. I usually walk away praying that they will have a change of heart, because most of these people will not listen to others trying to "preach" to them. They know it already. Lead a good clean life. Don't kill or steal. Go to heaven when you die. Period, is that right? Wrong!

Romans 4:4, tells us that you cannot earn your way into heaven by your good deeds. The only way to heaven is through the gift of salvation. We are not born with this gift of God's salvation we have to ask for it. That's the only stipulation.

Just believing in Jesus is not enough. The Bible tells us that even the demons of hell know Jesus.

Good deeds and believing are not enough. We need to ask for God to cleanse our heart and forgive us of our sins. We need to pause and ask him right now if we've not accepted him in the past. We should not continue going through each day wondering if we are going to heaven. We need to be sure!

People seem to think life comes with a two minute warning bell like some sports do. They just go about their business, until their warning bell goes off, then they will hurriedly ask Jesus' forgiveness. But life doesn't come with a warning bell.

I've heard other people say all they need is five minutes before they die to make things right. Well, that might be okay if they have a terminal condition that advances slowly. They may have time to decide when to make that decision. A person who is driving on the interstate and suddenly sees a tractor trailer crossing the center line after the driver has fallen asleep will not have time to ask forgiveness. If a person has a heart attack and passes away while asleep, he or she won't have an opportunity to ask forgiveness. I've known people who have left to go to the store for milk and have not made it back.

Let's face it. God is the only one who knows when our time will come to leave this life, and he is not telling.

Ask God to forgive you of your sins, then, find a good church to become involved in. This helps you to learn and grow in spiritual strength and knowledge. This strength and knowledge is what we need to prevent us from falling back into our old sinful ways.

As for the other people who are attending church, they are there for the same reason that we are; to support one another with taking one more step forward and then another.

Remember, it's not the healthy people who need to go to the doctor. It's the sick ones, the broken ones, the hurt ones. The ones you'll find in church. Hope to see you there.

❧ Hebrews 10:25

"Let us not give up meeting together, as some are in the habit of doing, but let us encourage one another"

3.
Fear

What are we afraid of? Maybe it's spiders or snakes. Maybe we're afraid to speak to a large crowd of people. Maybe we're just afraid of the dark.

There are definitely a lot of things to be afraid of in this life. Every day on the news, someone is murdered. There are natural disasters, such as floods, earthquakes, even tornadoes and hurricanes that crop up unexpectedly to destroy homes and businesses. There is illness, such as cancer that can rob people of their health. The list of possible fears is endless, and the list is different for each of us.

Most of the time, we are just afraid to trust God. We don't really trust him 100 percent of the time, do we? People will say "That's crazy! Of course I trust God!" Do we, 100 percent of the time, in every situation?

When God tells us to do something, do we automatically do it, trusting that God will provide us with his grace to get it done? Or do we back away from some situations because we are afraid? Do we keep questioning ourselves, saying surely God wouldn't want me to do that, would he?

Maybe he wants us to walk up and talk to a stranger. Maybe he wants us to stand up and give a testimony. Maybe he wants us to join a mission trip. Are we going to jump right into it, and do what God has put on our heart without question? Or are we going to say "I can't talk to that person, I don't even know them." Or "I'm sorry God, but I'm afraid to stand up in front of the church to give my testimony."

Recently, I had one of these conversations with God, regarding something he wanted to do in my life. I knew what he wanted, but I was telling him I was afraid, afraid of the change it would bring into my life, afraid of having to speak to a lot of people.

I will tell you exactly what God told me. He said "Then do it afraid." You see, God wasn't about to let me back out, and I wanted to be obedient to God. We all want to be obedient, and when God first brings up his plans for us, it's easy to say "Yes Lord."

Then what happens? After we've agreed, we start to have second thoughts. And as we move closer and closer to what God wants, we start to get butterflies, and we start to become anxious about it. We try to come up with ways that we can bargain to God, offering to do something else, if only he will let us off the hook about the thing we fear.

Do it afraid. We just have to forget all of our insecurities and step out. Step out in faith. God will be with us each step of the way, but he can't be with us if we don't take that first step. If we just stand rooted to the same spot and don't go anywhere, then we'll never accomplish anything.

Proverbs 3:6 "In everything acknowledge God and he will direct your steps." You see, we have to trust that if God is telling us to do something, then he will definitely be with us to help get it done.

I feel sure that Noah would have been afraid when God told him to build the ark, and gather the animals. Maybe, he would have been afraid of looking foolish for building a boat, when it hadn't rained before, but I believe that he did it afraid.

When Moses was chosen to lead the Israelites out of Egypt, he was afraid and insecure. If you were chosen for that chore, would you have been afraid? I know I would have been!

There are so many examples in the Bible, where God called regular people like you and me, and told them to do extraordinary things. Things that probably sounded strange to them at the time. I can truly believe that each of them were probably terrified. But they did it! And when they did it, they found that God was there with them. God was there with Daniel in the lion's den, with David facing the giant, and he's here with each of us also.

Fear is a lack of trust. Fear is thinking that we are all alone and vulnerable. We need to give that fear over to God. He knows we're afraid, and he will give us the strength we need. We just need to believe and trust in him.

We need to realize that no one has ever died from speaking to a crowd of people, or from talking to a stranger about Jesus. The person may have felt like it for the moment, but they didn't.

If God has laid something on our heart to do, we need to take a deep breath and just step out in faith, even if we have to do it afraid.

❧ Isaiah 41:10

"Do not fear for I am with you; do not be dismayed for I am your God. I will strengthen you and help you; I will uphold you with my righteous right hand."

4.
Thoughts

We've all seen a person with a physical handicap. We may have a family member with a physical handicap, or we may have one. Have we ever noticed that many of these people keep their heads lowered? I know that the majority of the time it is from their physical condition, either from the lack of muscle strength, or lack of coordination. Often, they need support devices, such as straps, belts, or collars to give them stability.

But, what if they are looking down because they are uncomfortable with the looks, and stares of others; or feel that they are being over looked, or ignored by other people around them.

Imagine if we put ourselves in that other person's spot. Even without the physical disability, haven't we all felt that we could not bring ourselves to raise our head to meet the stares of those around us?

We have often let Satan cripple our walk with God in this way. He has disabled us, maybe not physically, but mentally. When we feel like this, it is a sign that we have a handicapped mind set. Satan loves it when we feel this way. This is Satan's bondage over us, and we should not allow it.

We have all been in a group of people and felt that we were alone, or felt that we were different, and just did not belong. We have shut people out of our lives that God has tried to bring along beside us to help us. We have the support available to assist us to lift our heads, like family, friends, and of course Jesus, but we don't use them. They just remain useless at our side.

How did we get here? Most of the time, we have put ourselves here with our own insecurities and guilt over things we have done in the past. We feel ashamed. We might ask ourselves "how can I lift my head and look at other people after what I've done?" Whether it's true or not, we can sense that other person's condemnation of us.

Of course, Satan is leaning over our shoulder whispering these very things in our ear, but we can't see that it's him speaking, because we have our head down, and eyes downcast. We don't even glance up to see who's speaking. If we did, then we would know that it is Satan's lies

Remember that whatever it is in our past cannot be changed. We have to live with the knowledge that we did it; but we can remember that Jesus has forgiven us for it. If we have never asked for his forgiveness, we need to.

Sometimes, we will develop this handicap because of someone else and their collision with us. We are often so blindsided by the circumstances, that we do not realize how hurt we are until we cannot lift our heads. We become numb and paralyzed for a while, and usually we heal as a cripple.

Maybe it was a divorce, where a spouse just refused to try to work things out, or a child who has gotten into trouble with the cops. Maybe it was a family member who has made the wrong kind of name for themselves. Maybe it was a tragedy that struck, or a friend's betrayal.

Whatever it is, it has put us here, and we need help.

Luke 13:11, talks about the woman who had been bent over double for 18 years. Can you imagine 18 years of looking at the ground? Every day, all we would see is the dirt and dust on the sidewalks and the roads, the trash that people have thrown down, the empty bottles and cans, the cigarette butts, and gum wrappers. Sometimes we may even see the chewed, discarded gum itself.

We can't see the clouds, so we don't even know it's raining until we're getting wet. We haven't seen the sun shining, or how it glistens through the trees. And what about the trees, are they out in fall foliage? The beautiful red, gold, and orange leaves in the fall, we've missed them again, because we refuse to look up.

All the while, Satan is laughing at us as we stumble along, our eyes downcast, our shoulders bent under the weight, and we can't even see what we're about to run into. But God is watching it all.

Believe me God doesn't miss a thing, especially where his children are concerned. Even though we can't lift our heads, all we have to do is call to him, or maybe just lift one hand to reach out for him. Everyone else might be looking over top of us as they hurry by, but God is looking at us. And just like the woman in the book of Luke, he can't stand to see us suffering, and he will heal us. He will touch us and we will stand straight!

We need to say "Forget you Satan!" We are upright and walking tall next to Jesus. Look up because we are forgiven and healed. Because Jesus is with us, we're never alone or overlooked. My, has the sky always been that blue?

❧ Romans 5:5

"We are able to hold our heads high no matter what happens and know that all is well, for we know how dearly God loves us, and we feel this warm love everywhere within us because God has given us the Holy Spirit to fill our hearts with his love."

5.
Desires

Who are we when no one's looking? There is a country music song currently playing on the radio that is called "Who are you when I'm not looking?" The lyrics are about a man asking this question to the woman in his life. He wants to know what she does when she's all alone and he's not there with her. He wants to know how she is spending her time "when the door is locked and the window shades are down".

How do we spend our time alone? Especially at the end of the day, when we are home alone, or relaxing with just our family. It's so easy to act like a Christian when we are in a crowd of people. We can be on our best behavior when there are other people watching us. But who are we when we go home and "the door is locked and the window shades are down?"

Are we leading a double life? Would our close family be shocked at the good acting job we put on when we are at work or out with our friends? Would our friends be in disbelief, if they saw a hidden video of us, and saw how we spend our free time?

We have to remember that nothing is hidden from God. NOTHING!

Ecclesiates12:14 "God will judge us for everything we do, including every hidden thing, good or bad." We may think it's hidden, but God has seen it.

There was a very close relative of mine, who was the absolute nicest man you would ever want to meet. He would always be laughing, and he could tell such great stories. He also loved dogs, and would gather up strays that he found. Many times, I saw him give his last dollar to a friend, and then leave himself without money to get food, or even gas for his car.

This man was also hiding a secret that few other people knew. He would come home in the evenings, and abuse his wife and terrorize his kids. Many times, when I was young I saw his wife with bruises or a black eye. I'm sure that God did not approve of this. A man is to love and care for his wife, whether they are out in public together, or spending the evening at home.

Do we have something hidden, and we would just die, if other people found out about it?

Are we so frustrated at the end of the day that we go home, kick the dog, and beat our kids? Do we rant and rave at our spouse, and then put on a big smile to answer the door and chat with our neighbor?

Maybe we are in financial debt because we like to sneak off to the next town, where nobody recognizes us, and we spend the entire day playing the slot machines.

Maybe we're partying and drinking, and hooking up with other people on Saturday, but sitting in our same back row pew at church on Sunday.

Maybe we've developed an emotional connection with a co-worker, and we're contemplating an affair, or maybe we have already started one, sneaking off for hidden rendezvous' in another part of town where our car won't be recognized.

We may think that we are getting away with these things because nobody saw us. But can we be sure they didn't? We still go to work every day, look our co-workers in the eye, and pretend we are normal. We pretend that we are just like them, but maybe they are doing these same things.

We may think that we have gotten away with it, but we didn't. Our actions might not be brought to light while we are still here on earth, but God is an all seeing, all knowing God. We forgot about him, didn't we? He never forgets about us, and because he can't forget us, he is keeping watch on us ALL THE TIME!

He knows what we're planning to do, even before we do. Our neighbors might not have seen our car parked where it shouldn't be, but God knew we were going there before we even left.

We can't act like a devil on Saturday night, and then pretend to be a saint on Sunday morning.

1 Corinthians 10:21 "You cannot drink from the cup at the Lord's table and at Satan's table too." We have to choose if we will follow God's ways, whether the world is watching or not.

We will always have the two desires, one to do good things for Christ, and our own fleshly desires and temptations to do wrong, fighting inside of us for control. We will never be free from these pressures.

We need to remember, the next time our flesh is screaming for us to do something wrong, and the devil is whispering in our ear "Go ahead, nobody's looking", that God is always watching.

✌ Romans 13:12-13

"So quit the evil deeds of darkness and put on the armor of right living, as we who live in the daylight should! Be decent and true in everything you do so that all can approve your behavior."

6.
Priorities

We need to get our priorities in order, but what is our priority? Maybe it is our family, our home, our career, or even our children. After all, these are important to us, right? Now, where does God fall in that list? Do we squeeze him in once a year at Easter, or Christmas? Maybe it is for one hour, once a week, on Sunday.

Are we in constant conversations with him throughout the day, while we do the laundry, or grocery shopping, or do we only remember him when we're in trouble? God should always be first in our lives. We need to remember the 1st Commandment "You shall have no other God before me." There are a lot of things that we would not classify as gods, but we elevate them to the same level of importance as God.

These things become idols in our lives, every bit the same as the carved idols from the Old Testament. These idols can be another person, or a thing; it can be anything that takes the place of God in our life.

Maybe it's that job of ours, where we spend 40-50 hours or more a week, the one that we feel no one else can do but us.

Maybe it's the car that we are constantly polishing and waxing, or the old muscle car that we take to the parades and the car shows.

Maybe it's our house, the one we can't stop cleaning, until we could eat off of the floors. The same house, with a manicured lawn, that could be on the cover of a magazine.

Maybe it's the spouse, or the boyfriend/girlfriend, the one that we can't stop worrying over when they are out of our sight; the same one that we are constantly fussing over, when they are with us. Could it be the new baby that we're always hovering over, and running to when it makes the slightest noise in their sleep; the same one that we're neglecting our other relationships for, such as our husband or our other children?

Now let's delve a little deeper.

Could our idols be an addiction to drugs or alcohol? Some people have to have it, and will do anything to get it.

Money, of course is a big idol for a lot of people. Some people are constantly worried about making another dollar; many people won't even help their neighbor anymore, without expecting something in return.

Many things can fall under this category of idols, so we have to be careful, and really ask God on a daily basis to search our heart, and show us what we have exalted to his level.

Next, is pride in our own abilities, or accomplishments; now, we have exalted ourselves above God. We can do NOTHING apart from God, so whatever we have just accomplished was done through God, and the entire glory is his, not ours.

Let's even explore grief. I know that grief is a natural process, and like you, I have loved and lost people that were precious to me. What is not natural, is allowing God to walk us through the natural healing and grief process, but instead we become angry, embittered, and continue to grieve without end. We have now idolized that person, and our grief, to an exalted level. What we are saying is this particular person, and what we lost, were so important that we cannot accept God's healing touch. We are saying that God is not strong enough to remove the pain we are in.

There are many stories throughout the Old Testament, regarding little children being sacrificed to false idols. Sons and daughters that were completely innocent; these were children of peasants, as well as kings. Children, who were trusting adults to care for them, and instead were thrown into the fire and killed needlessly, sacrificed to an idol. A fake god! What a waste of a precious life.

Think about the idols of our day and time that we just looked at. Sure, they aren't made of carved pieces of wood or golden images of bronze, or silver, but they are idols just the same. I've given some ideas of the most common idols that God has shown me for today's society. I'm sure there are many more examples; but what bothers me the most is that the little children are still being sacrificed to idols. They are still being burned, and destroyed, by our search for "our god", the only thing, that will bring us happiness, and fulfillment. In the meantime, the children are being destroyed.

How many children are home alone, because their parents are worshiping the idol called the corporate ladder; or are starved, and neglected, even prostituted, for parents who have a drug or alcohol addiction?

How about the ones abused by the mother's new boyfriend that she refuses to live without?

Juvenile hall and foster care are full of the emotionally, and physically, destroyed children who were sacrificed by the idol worshiping adults in their lives.

Let's get our priority straight. God is our priority. Our family is our priority. Don't be an idol worshipper. Our God is a jealous God, and he will share his place with nothing, and no one.

ઇ 1 Samuel 1:27

"For this child, I have prayed."

7.
Judging

The bible says "Judge not lest you be judged." How many of us judge other people around us? All of us do, I know. And we're not choosey in who we judge. Foe, family or friend, they all come under our radar as fair game.

We judge what people wear, what they say, what they do, or don't do. We tell ourselves, that we would never do what they do, so by our standards, we're right and they're wrong. But the world doesn't care about my standards, or your standards, only God's standards. God is our judge and jury, and if it's right, okay. If it's not right, the Holy Spirit will convict us, and one day we will have to answer for it on Judgment Day.

When we judge another person ourselves, we have convicted them of the crime, sentenced them, and hung them. We are now acting like an old time vigilante; we didn't wait for justice to run its course, we have already found the other person guilty.

After all, the person was definitely wrong, weren't they? We feel that they should have known better than to wear that outfit out in public, or to date that type of a man; and what were they thinking when they styled their hair like that.

I don't know the answer, let's check the rule book. The problem is that we don't have a rule book for a lot of the silly stuff that people are judged on. But, we do have the rule book that God left us. It's called the Bible.

It tells us how we should talk, and how to behave in certain situations, so that we stay within God's correct guidelines. It tells us the correct way to handle our finances, our marriage, and even how to raise our children.

If we don't follow the rules, then that is between us and God, not the nosy neighbor down the street.

There are a lot of little details that are not in the Bible because I think that God was not concerned with them. Things that he says we may choose, like how we cut our hair, how we want to style it, even whether we should wear sneakers with that outfit, or pumps. God doesn't care about fashion trends, as long as we are keeping within the lines of modesty that he set for women, go wild.

If we have a favorite belt that we love, wear it every day if we want, it will cause the people around us to go crazy, but God doesn't care about it. If we want our hair cut short or long, maybe even dyed pink, okay, it is just hair. It is our hair, and our choice. God does not say that we have to have our hair a certain length or style. He doesn't care if we wear stripes and plaids together, or white after Labor Day. That's our choice, and even though the world around us may judge us on these things, and the fashion police will remark on our lack of fashion sense, we are not outside of God's obedience. But the people who are doing the censoring are.

By judging other people, they are saying that God is not able to handle the situation. That God isn't strong enough to bring that other person into line if they need it.

Now that is a sin. We are not to question God's judgment, even if we feel he is not properly correcting someone who is doing wrong. That is none of our business. That is between God and that other person. You see, people may be looking at us and thinking the same thing about the things that we are doing. They may be wondering why God has not stepped in and corrected us.

We do not need to worry because God knows what he's doing. He can handle the situation. He will correct each of us as we need it according to his perfect timing and in his perfect way.

Life is short, let's stop worrying about what everyone else is doing, or not doing, and enjoy it. God has everything under control.

❧ Romans 14:10

"You have no right to criticize your brother or look down on him. Remember, each of us will stand personally before the Judgment seat of God."

8.
Laughter

Have we had our laugh for today? Have we ever been so stressed out while doing something, and then, all of a sudden, something will happen that strikes us as funny, and we just start to laugh? Don't we always feel better afterward, more able to handle the task at hand?

I've even heard frustrated people say "I don't know whether to laugh or cry." Why is that?

Both of these emotional responses can act as a big stress reliever. They both release tension, and can work on the soul as well. A good healthy cry will actually cleanse the soul. We just seem to bring all of the pent up emotion out of the deep part of our soul. But a hearty laugh seems to fill up our soul. A good, healthy, gut busting laugh is said to be the best kind of medicine for our body and soul. When we laugh, we just feel good all over, don't we? Doesn't the day just seem to be brighter when we can get in a laugh or two; it puts us in a calmer, more carefree frame of mind.

We are even able to deal with each other better when we are able to laugh together. It helps to create a bond with each other, and makes us look forward to spending time together.

Sometimes, we just take each other and ourselves too seriously. We need to learn to laugh at things. After all, most of the time we can't change the circumstances anyway, so we might as well lighten up, and put a different perspective on it. There's no use to go around with a sour looking face and attitude. That won't change anything, in fact it will usually just make it worse, because now we've made everyone around us just as miserable as we are, and who wants to deal with a sourpuss all day? I sure don't. We're only on this earth for a short time, so we should make the most of it, and try to enjoy it.

My mother in law once confided to me that my father in law thinks that she and I are sometimes a little odd, because when we are together, we always find something amusing to laugh about. Sometimes we start to giggle like a couple of school girls. Now, my dear mother in law is in her early seventy's and I'm closer to fifty than I am to forty, so I guess people expect us to act our age; but we have just learned to enjoy ourselves and be young at heart.

When the situation calls for it, we can be as determined, focused, and serious as the next person, but we don't need to be like that in every situation.

I think even God likes a good laugh now and then, don't you? I have had situations where I am positive that God has a sense of humor, just because of the ridiculously easy or humorous way, that he will work problems out for us in our lives.

We need to look for the humor in our situations, believe me, it's usually there.

Now, God does not want us to disrespect ourselves and talk down about ourselves, but we can find, and share, the humor in a lot of our everyday mistakes. After all, we are only human, so we make quite a few.

I have known people who will continuously beat themselves up over some of the stupid things that they have done. As long as nobody was seriously harmed, we can laugh about it and go on. A lot of our family and friends are making the same kind of crazy mistakes that we are.

We don't need to point fingers and try to embarrass someone else about their mistakes, because I can guarantee you that sooner or later we will make one too. Maybe even more silly than the other person's mistake was. We should learn to lighten up and laugh at ourselves.

When we are able to laugh at ourselves that will give other people around us the permission to join in, and wouldn't that be a joyous sound to hear everyone laughing. God enjoys seeing us having a good time and getting along. Remember, laugh and the world laughs with you, maybe even God too.

❧ Proverbs 17:22

"A merry heart doeth good like a medicine, but
a broken spirit drieth the bones."

9.
Love

God has a message us. He loves us. Yes, it's true. He loves us, isn't that wonderful! He made us, so he knows us, and he loves us. He has counted the hairs on our head, he keeps our tears in a jar, he knew us when we were still in the womb, and he loves us. He knows our comings and goings, and wants nothing more than to show us how much he loves us.

Maybe we think we are not worthy of his love, or we don't know how he could love us because of the bad things we've done in the past. Well, guess what, he already knows! He knows what we've done, what we've said, and even what we have thought, and he still loves us!

Have we asked for forgiveness of those past sins? It's simple, just confess what they are to God, and tell him how sorry we are. Now those sins are in the past and behind us, but maybe we shouldn't put them behind us, we should actually lay them all at Jesus' feet. We can let him put our past sinful ways behind him, and then we won't be able to turn around and pick them up again. Now we have to go through Jesus if you try to get them back.

Sometimes, we may still feel unworthy, even after we've confessed our sins, and received forgiveness. The hardest part is that we have to BELIEVE we are forgiven. We have to stop worrying about our sins, they're gone, vanished, forgiven, under the blood, because Jesus took them, now we have to believe it.

Our human, self-condemning nature can't stop God's forgiveness, but it can keep us from feeling that we are forgiven and from believing it. This is why so many people continue with the same roller coaster ride of sin. They will sin, then ask for forgiveness, but then either they don't believe it, or they can't comprehend it, so they say, "what the heck, I might as well do it again."

Now God, as our father is waiting patiently at the exit gate to that roller coaster ride of sin, and like any father, his eyes are on us as we go around and around. He's just waiting until we are so sick of the ups and downs, and twists and turns, that we could puke. He is waiting for us to cry out, "I've had enough, get me off this ride!" Then, he will take our hand, and lead us away from that ride, with our tear streaked face, upset stomach, and wobbly knees. We will look up at him and say, "I'm sorry, I know you told me not to ride that roller coaster, you told me it wasn't fun." And he will smile, and squeeze our hand as we continue to walk away, and he will say "I know, I forgive you and I still love you."

But, as we walk away, with our head down, there's a little inkling in the back of our head saying "He forgives you? Who are you kidding? He can't forgive you! He's God, he's perfect, and look what you just did!" Now the devil has what he wants, he knows he has no control over God's children, but he can plant a seed of doubt. He will give us the idea that we are not forgiven, and then stand back and laugh when we take that idea, no matter how wrong it is, and run with it. And where do we run? Hopefully not back to our sinful past, and that crazy roller coaster.

We need to run to God! We need to run to our father! What father wouldn't comfort and protect his children when they are threatened or scared. He loves us. He has forgiven us, and we must believe it!

We know all of our sins, and our weaknesses, and why God shouldn't love us. Every one of us thinks that the person next to us can't be as messed up as we have been. And why do we have such trouble believing that God can love the people we perceive as good, and also those we perceive as bad? Because that is how we are. We tend to love people according to how they act, but that is human love, and God isn't human.

Do we still have trouble really believing and accepting how much God loves us? Do we say "but I can't just make myself feel like God loves me."

Belief is not a feeling. It's a choice. We all have plenty of days when we don't feel loved, or lovely, but we can choose to take God at his word. To not believe is a sin. You see, the Bible tells us God loves us, and if we can't believe that part of his word, we don't believe any of it.

God sent his son to die for us. Do we think he would do that if he didn't love us?

1 John 4:10 "It was not our love of him, but his love for us that sent Christ to die for us."

John 17:23 "How much has God loved you, as much as he loved his son."

God's love made the world, and God nailed down his love on the cross. Now, can we imagine the grief God must feel because of our unbelief, even after all he's done for us? God is pure love, and there is not one time when we pray, and tell the Lord that we love him, when he has not already told us first; so the next time we are praying, we just need to say, "Thank you Lord- I love you too!"

ꙮ Romans 7:24-25

"My new life tells me to do right, but the old nature that is still inside me loves to sin. Who will free me from my slavery to this deadly lower nature? Thank God! It has been done by Jesus Christ our Lord. He has set me free."

10.
Marriage

Did you know that the divorce rate in the USA is 50 percent? This means that one half of all the people that get married this year will become divorced. That's a huge number, and it only gets worse. 67 percent of second marriages, and 74 percent of third marriages, also end in divorce.

How did we get to this? God does not want divorce. He sanctified marriage between two people of the opposite sex and blessed this union. We need to remember these words from our marriage vows, "What God has brought together, let no man put asunder." Let NO MAN put asunder. That includes our self!

These end times, that I believe we are living in, make it so easy to get divorced; and divorce is so commonplace, nobody blinks an eye at someone who is on their third, fourth, or even fifth marriage. The children in school, with both parents still living at home, and without a step-parent, or step-sibling in the picture, are truly the minority today.

We need to get ourselves, and our marriages, back in line with God's principles before we also end up as a statistic. How do we do that? We invite God back into the mix. Our marriage should be us, our spouse, and God. Ecclesiastes 4:12 "A triple braided cord is not easily broken." That third cord is God; we need to let him strengthen our union.

We leave our parents and become one with our spouse. This other person is now the single most priority in our life next to God. Their welfare is now our responsibility. Our spouse comes before our job, our friends, or our parents. Even above our future children.

So many marriages end up broken after the children come along, usually because one of the spouses will elevate the child into the place of importance that the other spouse should occupy. They become so focused on that child, they tend either to ignore the spouse, or become overprotective of that child to the point that the child will not listen to the other spouse.

We need to ALWAYS stand united against the storms of life, whether it is an issue with child rearing, finances, or whatever else comes our way. We need to stand firm side by side to face it, or fight it, whichever the case might be. A house divided will always fall!

Men are to love their wives as they love themselves. That means they should always treat her kindly, be gentle, never harsh, and always be ready to forgive. They should not criticize, or speak degradingly, to her or about her to others. Proverbs 31:10 "If you can find a truly good wife, she is worth more than precious gems, and if she is treated as such she will truly sparkle and light up your life."

Women, we are called to respect our husbands at all times, whether we feel they truly deserve respect, according to their actions, or not. We also should not criticize or speak ill of our spouse. God has placed the men as the leaders, and the head of the household. Now, this does not mean that we can't make decisions, remember, marriage is a united front, a team effort. We should talk decisions and problems through with each other, and pray about them, but the Bible clearly states that the final decision regarding the family falls to the husband. Wives, if we feel strongly that he is making a wrong decision, we can still approach him about it, and voice our concerns in a respectful manner without nagging. In the end, we should abide by his final decision on the matter. God will reward us for this.

Sometimes, things will happen in life to cause the spouse's roles to be reversed. Maybe due to illness, or a disability that now limits one of the spouses, and that is okay, but the commandment of the wife to respect the husband, and for the husband to show love to the wife, should always be followed.

The home that we make together should always be a safe haven for each of us to be ourselves, and to let ourselves be vulnerable, without the risk of attack or ridicule by the other. It should be a place to find comfort and refuge from the outside storms of this world. Don't let the little every day, mundane things destroy our marriage. Make time for each other. God has given us this person to spend the rest of our life with. They are a gift from God, so we should treasure them.

☙ Hebrews 13:4

"Honor your marriage and its vows, and be pure; for God will surely punish all those who are immoral or commit adultery."

11.
Neighbors

One of the ten commandants is to "Love thy neighbor", but who is our neighbor? I know that our neighbor does not necessarily mean the person living in the closest house to us. Our neighbor is also the person in the next cubicle at work, and the person that we stand next to in line at the grocery store. These are all our neighbors.

Do we love them? We don't even know them, do we? I'll be honest, I live in a duplex, in the borough of a small town, and have other houses that surround me on each side, but I can't tell you the names of all the people on the street. I can tell you the names of the ones on each side of me, and only the first name of the guy across the street.

It's not that I don't care about them. If they needed something, I would try to help them, but life is so busy that we can't take time to chit chat with our neighbors. We wave and smile as we see each other getting into our cars, or bringing groceries into the house, but that's about the extent of it.

Are our neighbors Christians, Seven Day Adventist, Muslim, Hindu, or Atheist? We don't know, do we?

Are you like me, and watch America's Most Wanted every week, praying that our neighbors are not on there? It's scary anymore.

When I was a kid growing up, I lived in the borough of an even smaller town, but of course it seemed big to me at the time. But I knew the name of the person, who lived in every single house, the whole way up and down the entire street.

Things seemed so simple when I was young. People spoke to each other, and they sat on their porch, and watched as the kids played in the yard. Parents didn't have to worry about us kids. They knew that the other parents would keep an eye on us, and send us home if we got out of line. The same way our parents were doing with their children. Children actually played outside all day long. We knew to be home for supper, and again when the street lamps came on, then we would yell "Ollie, Ollie, Oxen Free", the game would be over, time to go home.

Kids don't play outside like that anymore. It seems like my five grandchildren never go outside to play. They listen to their IPods, play their Wiis, or lie on their beds and talk to all of their friends on their cell phones. We didn't have all that when I was young. We played softball, kickball, and hide-n go seek; if we wanted to talk to our friends, we rang their doorbell, and asked their mother if they could come outside.

Kids don't want to walk down the street to see their friends nowadays. It's too far for them. So we hop in the car, with gas prices at almost $4.00 a gallon, and drive our kids two or three blocks to their friend's house, and then they'll call us to come get them again.

I'm not putting anyone down for this behavior because I have five grand-kids, and I occasionally will get pulled into this behavior also. I watch my daughters, running one way and then the other, taking the kids to after school activities, or to meet a friend, and it makes me tired.

I know how our behavior came to this, and there seems to be no way to fix it until Jesus comes and says that it is finished. It all started with kids being kidnapped and found outside of town, raped and murdered. It started with the serial murderers giving young girls a ride, and then they are never heard from again. It's the homes being robbed, while the people are in bed asleep.

We look at each other with caution. I don't know you, and you don't know me, and I'm not going to let you get close enough to harm me or my family.

Now, Jesus knows who our neighbors are. It doesn't matter if it's the atheist next door. He might not know Jesus, but Jesus knows him. And there will come a time when they will formally meet face to face.

Romans 14:11 "Every knee shall bow and every tongue confess that I am Lord." It doesn't say only the Christians' knees will bow, or that only those saved will confess.

It says "EVERY KNEE WILL BOW, AND EVERY TONGUE CONFESS."

We are still called to love our neighbors, each of them, regardless of their current religious views. We are to show them kindness when we can, help them if they need it, and show them God, even if they won't let us tell them about him. Don't worry, they will eventually be introduced.

❧ James 2:8

"You must love and help your neighbors just as
much as you love and take care of yourself."

12.
Guidance

1 Corinthians 10:29 asks an important question "Why must I be guided and limited by what someone else thinks?"

Does it matter what other people think about our walk with God? Are we responsible to these people around us?

1 Corinthians 11:3 reminds us that a wife is responsible to her husband, her husband is responsible to Christ, and Christ is responsible to God. Each of us as individuals, are also responsible to Christ, for both our actions and our spoken words.

I believe that in many ways, we are to be guided and limited by those around us. We are to be examples of our walk with Christ, so that we can lead those around us to him. This means that we must be conscious of our speech and our actions at all times. We can't be constantly, and intentionally sinning, and still expect people to follow us.

We should be open to opportunities at home, or in the workplace, to share the gospel with others, but we must also lead by example. If we are going to share the gospel with others, we need to make sure that we are living right, or how can we expect to be taken seriously? Remember, if we're going to talk the talk, we must walk the walk!

We are told in the bible to help the younger men and women around us; but will they want our help if we appear to be a hypocrite? We can't be partying and drinking on Saturday night, and then think we are doing good by going to church on Sunday morning.

We all fall into sin at one time or another. Nobody, but Christ, was ever able to get through this life without sin. When we fall, God will place someone beside us to help pick us up, and dust us off, and see that we are able to continue our walk again. Sometimes, we are that person that God is placing in someone's life to pick them up. Sometimes we are there for just a season, sometimes for a lifetime; either way, we walk away changed by what we saw, and by what that other person was thinking. So again, we can be guided by someone else's thinking, and in turn, that person can be guided and changed by ours.

I believe also that God wants to have a close relationship with each of us, and that is what we were created for. Everyone's walk or journey through life and their relationship with God is different. My relationship with God is different from yours, and someone else's may be different than both of ours.

Things might happen in our life to change our thinking, and our relationship with God. Some people were not brought up in a Christian home, or have not had the opportunity to go to church, or Sunday school as a child, maybe this has given them a slower start at finding Jesus. Others, who were brought up in a church, might have a closer relationship with God, one that was founded in childhood. Some people will even stray away from God, and then later return. Maybe some become so embittered with the circumstances of life, that they make the next right turn away from God, and hit the gas to go as fast, and as far away from him as they can. What they forget, is that when they are sitting on the side of the road, with no more gas in their car, steam billowing out from under the hood, and one flat tire, is that Jesus will be there to give them a ride in his tow truck and to tow their junk away as well.

We've all been here, haven't we? Will we accept the offer, or will we roll up the windows, lock the doors, and stare straight ahead, ignoring Jesus' tap on our window?

Whether we decide to accept is nobody else's decision but our own. Regardless of anyone else's opinion, we are the only one able to unlock the door and get out of the car. Nobody can do it for us. And where-ever we go from there, whether we accept the ride, or hitch hike later, is up to us. Jesus will not force us to accept. You see, our decision is a personal one. Regardless of what people say or think, the decision has to come from us.

Whether we are a preacher's son, or a mechanics daughter, everyone has to eventually make this decision on their own. Nobody can do this for us.

Once the decision is made to follow God, we need to start a relationship with him, and ask him daily to help us to learn more about him. Don't listen to our old friends who tell us that he's not real, or that we don't need him. Don't let others guide us in that direction. Ask Jesus to draw us close and place other people in our life to help us, he will. Remember, we may need the help now, and in return God may use us later in someone else's life.

And we shouldn't allow people to judge us regarding how many chapters we read daily in our bible, or how much time we spend in prayer. These are personal issues between us and God, and they should not be dependent upon what other people think is right for us.

What will we choose today....Jesus' way or the highway?

❧ Romans 6:16

"Don't you realize that you can choose your own master? You can choose sin and death, or else choose obedience and life."

13.
Parents

Growing up, our parents are the most important people in our lives, aren't they? I can remember running to mom or dad when I would fall and skin my knee, which seemed to be all the time, when I was a kid. They would clean the scrape and put ointment on it, and back outside I'd go, usually to do it all over again.

But that didn't matter. It didn't matter how many times I fell and scraped my knees, I always knew that I could run back into the house crying, and one of my parents would be there to clean me up, give me a hug, and tell me it was okay. That's what parents do. That's their job. God gave us these parents to take care of us throughout our lives.

We can't choose our parents, and what they will be like, any more than we can choose the baby that we will have. We can't say, "Okay, I'm going to have a baby boy with blonde hair and blue eyes, and I want him to grow up to be 6 ft. tall, and be an engineer when he grows up." It can't be done. We get what we get, because that's how God felt that it should be according to his divine plan.

What God has said, is that we should honor our mother and father so that we may have a long life. This apparently is something God felt very strongly about, as he decided to add on "so you will live a long life", at the end of "Honor thy mother and father." He's saying do this, or else he will take us out of the picture all together.

When we're little kids, our parents are everything. Then into the teenage years, we tend to pull away from our parents, after all we're teenagers, we think we know it all and they don't know anything. This is a normal part of spreading our wings in preparation to leave the nest. We need to learn some independence, but we need to make sure that we don't take it too far.

After we've made a few errors, and mom and dad has baled us out of a few scrapes, we start to realize that maybe we didn't know it all, don't we?

Now, just like with our Heavenly Father, our earthly parents won't totally desert us. They are there for us, and always will be, as long as we can humble ourselves to admit that we need them, and that we can't do everything on our own, like we thought. Of course our friends can't help us, they are in the same boat because they've got parents too.

The main thing we need to keep in mind is that our parents are human, just like us. We may have thought of them as superhuman, until we got to about age ten, but they're not; and because they are human, they are going to make mistakes as they raise us to adulthood, just like we will make mistakes as we raise their grandchildren.

Those of us that were raised in a less than perfect home need to learn to put aside our past hurts that we feel came from our parents. After all, they were trying to get through life the same way we are, juggling jobs, houses, and relationships. It's not easy. Life is not easy by any means, and if we can't give forgiveness, honor and respect to the parents who raised us, who should get it?

I hear about kids from broken homes, whose parents are divorced, and usually in these cases, one of the parents always come out as the bad guy. Maybe the divorce came as a result of someone's infidelity, maybe there was even abuse involved, maybe even abuse toward the children in the family, or maybe one of the parents just walked out of the picture and disappeared.

Whatever the scenario, we are still called to honor our parents, whether they are our birth parents, step parents, foster parents, or adoptive parents.

We need to forgive our parents for their mistakes, and pray that one day our children will forgive us for ours. We need to show them the respect that is called for, and if they need our help, we need to help them.

Lastly, I think honoring them also means not bringing up all of their mistakes that we feel were made while raising us; not in an accusatory manner to them directly, or to other family members and friends. If our parents are no longer alive, the same still applies. We should honor their name by speaking respectfully about them to others, and by letting go of any lasting resentment harbored toward them.

We should ask God to show us areas where we are dishonorable, than we need to ask for his forgiveness. After all, I want to live a long life, don't you?

❧ Hebrews 12:10-11

"Our earthly fathers trained us for a few brief years, doing the best for us that they knew how, but God's correction is always right and for our best good, that we may share his holiness. Being punished isn't enjoyable while it is happening- it hurts! But afterwards we can see the result, a quiet growth in grace and character."

14.
Problems

It happened again didn't it? Someone, or something, just messed up our whole day. Doesn't it seem like some days, it just doesn't pay for us to get out of bed? We've all had those days, haven't we? They seem to occur almost every day. Just like in the following example, you know the ones I'm talking about.

It's the kind of day where we're awakened during the night with a bad thunderstorm, only to wake up late the next morning, because the power went out during the night, and our alarm clock didn't go off.

Now, we're rushing to get the kids ready, but the faster we push them to get ready, the slower they go. Then, we can't find the keys to our car, and the cell phone's dead because we forgot to put it on the charger last night.

On the way to drop the kids off at school, we remember that we forgot to feed the dog and let him out; now we'll be worried all day about the mess on the floor we'll find when we get home.

We finally get to work, only to find our boss waiting to speak with us on the one day that we're ten minutes late. Somehow, we just knew he wouldn't be in a meeting, or miss our entrance today, didn't we?

We have no time for lunch, the phones are ringing off the hook, the copier is jammed, and the fax machine just ran out of ink. Oh yeah, it's one of those days alright!

After we pick up the kids, it's time for soccer practice, and homework; now the kids are fighting, and as we go to straighten them out the smoke detector starts going off! Oh no, we forgot about supper while we were playing referee!

Of course, hubby is on the couch watching the six o'clock news, and oblivious to the house falling in around him. What us women wouldn't give for one day of that selective hearing that some men have.

Now, it's time for dishes, and baths, and finishing the laundry, until finally, bedtime! Guess who's waiting to finally get some of our attention, and maybe even a little romance? We tell him, "Don't even think about it!" Now his feelings are hurt, and we're both sleeping back to back, without even a good night kiss.

Does this sound like our life? I know it sounds like mine. The problems might not be identical, but we all have them, just one problem, or another, to throw us off track for the day. We don't know why things like this happen, they just happen.

James 1:2 "Is your life full of difficulties? Then be happy." Did he really say that we should be happy? He's got to be kidding! "For when the way is rough, your patience has a chance to grow." Believe me, when I say that there are a lot of times when my patience is in short supply.

"So let it grow and don't try to squirm out of your problems. For when your patience is finally in full bloom, then you will be ready for anything, strong in character, full and complete." Strong in character and ready for anything, that's what Christ wants from us. He wants us to have a strong character, and be ready to work the harvest. How can we come along side someone to help them, if we've never went through any troubles ourselves?

We can only learn compassion if we've been on the receiving end of it before; otherwise, we might be able to speak the right words, but the true feelings aren't there to back it up.

1 Peter 1:6-7, "There is wonderful joy ahead, even though the going is rough for a while down here. These trials are only to test your faith, to see whether or not it is strong and pure."

There's that word again. Strong. These trials are to make us strong, just like gold that is heated, and purified by fire. God wants us to pass these tests so that we become pure, and strong in our faith, and so we can be used by him. And just like the bible story of Shadrach, Meshach, and

Abednego, we can walk through the fiery furnace and know that God is with us every step of the way.

☙ Psalms 119: 49-50

"Never forget your promises to me your servant for they are my only hope, they give me strength in all my troubles."

15.
Purpose

There's a great wave of spiritual soul searching going on. People are trying to find their purpose in life. They just want to know what we're here for, what life is all about, and why were we created.

So many people have this longing to know where to go from here, and what the future holds. People just jump from job to job, trying to find some fulfillment in their life; fulfillment that they think their job should be supplying.

People go to psychics, and fortune tellers, and spend hard earned money trying to get the answers to their questions. Self-help books sell out at bookstores, as people try to find a cure for the vague, restlessness that is their constant companion.

Some people change spouses like they do their underwear, just because the other person was no longer able to give them the satisfaction, and fulfillment that they needed. Other people are constantly changing houses, or cars, in search of something that will make them happy.

We might find some short term satisfaction in these things, but nothing that will last for the long term. Why? Because our life's purpose is not to have the biggest, or the best of everything; and it's not to have a high paying, stress ulcer causing job, or a mansion on the hill.

No matter how many times we divorce and remarry, we would never find the perfect spouse who can fulfill our every need. Our kids will not be perfect; they will get dirty, get noisy, and occasionally get the bad report cards from school.

But you know what? That's okay. We will go to bed tonight, and get up tomorrow, just like we did yesterday. We'll fix our meals, and take care of our families, and go to our jobs if we have one. We don't need to see a psychic, or to read our horoscope to know what's coming tomorrow. Tomorrow will be just like today, but that's okay too, because this is our purpose in life.

No, it's not glamorous, and a lot of days it's not easy, but it's what we're here to do. We are to take care of each other, to be a good steward over what God has given to us, and to have a relationship with Our Maker.

We are called to be fair and just, in our dealings with each other, and to help those that need us. Micah 6:8 "He has told you what he wants, and this is all it is, to be fair and just and merciful, and to walk humbly with your God."

Doesn't that sound a lot easier than rushing around for answers like we have been doing? All of the self-help books that we've read, and all the people we've asked have not done us any good. All along, God had the answer. After all, he is our Creator, so he is the best one to tell us what we were created for, right?

How simple it is. We can finally relax and just enjoy our lives because now we have found our purpose in life. Now, we can stop searching, and just fulfill our true purpose; and what happens when we can finally relax, and our minds are at rest? We find peace.

Peace, knowing that we are where God wants us to be, and that we are doing what God wants us to do. Now we can have peace knowing that this is our life's purpose. The other stuff, like our jobs, and where we should live to raise our kids, will all fall into place as long as we continue to walk humbly with God.

God will direct our steps and set our feet on a firm foundation. He is that foundation. As long as we are fulfilling our purpose in life, God will lead us through the twists and turns of this life until our purpose, and our journey is finished. Then, as we stand before the throne, God can say "Well done, welcome home!"

❧ Hebrews 13:8

"Jesus Christ is the same yesterday, today, and forever,
so do not be attracted by strange new ideas, your
spiritual strength comes as a gift from God."

16.
Respect

R-E-S-P-E-C-T! What does it really mean to us?

Aretha Franklin demanded it. Our parents demanded it from us, and in turn we demand it from our children. But what is it?

The encyclopedia says respect is "a positive feeling of esteem for a person or entity." In other words, our actions and our speech should both show, and reflect the positive esteem that we feel.

An example of this is someone who has respect for their native country is not going to burn its flag or try to terrorize it in some way.

In the same regard we would not curse, degrade or harm our parents, or any other relation or person that we have respect (and therefore high esteem) for.

Now we have gotten an idea about respect. We know what it is. We know who should get it, and some ways we should try to show it.

We want to show respect to our parents and grandparents, our president, and our country; but mostly, we want to show respect to our Lord. He is our Maker, the maker of heaven and earth. God, his son Jesus, and the Holy Spirit, this is the trinity, and they are all one and the same. If we show disrespect to one, then we've disrespected them all.

Now, if we respect God, then we also must respect his creations such as the earth, and all things in it, even ourselves. That's right, we need to respect ourselves. It is called having self-respect.

We do not belong to ourselves. We belong to God. We were made for God alone, and bought with a price.

1 Corinthians 6:19 tells us that our body is the home of the Holy Spirit that lives within us and our own body does not belong to us. Verse 20 says that God bought us with a great price and so we need to use every part of our body to give glory back to God, because he is the true owner.

Now, how exactly should we be using our bodies in a respectful manner?

For starters, we need to lead a moral life. There are specific things that the bible tells us are forbidden, and we need to abide by his word. We truly cannot be living an immoral life, and still be pointing the way to Jesus. Would we follow a thief or a drunkard? Would we trust that what they were telling us was true? I don't think so.

There are also a lot of things that we do that Jesus did not say no to, but we still have to be careful, because even though we are allowed to do them, they can get such a grip on us that we can't easily stop or control ourselves.

Take food for instance, God has given us food because he knows we need it, but this doesn't mean that we should eat more than we need. We have to remove food from the elevated place it holds in our lives.

Sexual sin is another way we disrespect our bodies. God did not make us for this purpose. Yes, he gave us sex as a way to populate the earth within the confines of marriage, but the Lord wants us to fill our bodies with him. We need to realize that our bodies are members of Christ. When two people are joined in sex, they become as one, so would you join Christ with a sinful sexual partner, such as in a homosexual relationship, or with a prostitute, or even that drunken one night stand? No other sin affects the body as this one does.

James 3:5-6 says "The tongue is a small thing, but what enormous damage it can do. It is full of wickedness, and it can poison every part of the body. The tongue can turn our whole lives into a blazing flame of destruction and disaster." AMEN!

Wow, I think we have all been there with this one. How many relationships are destroyed every day because of the tongue? Remember, once it leaves the tongue those words can never be brought back. We can apologize all we want later, but the damage has already been done.

That goes the same for ourselves, we can either build ourselves up, or tear ourselves down, with our own tongue.

How many times have we told someone how stupid we are, how we are just too fat, too thin, or not good enough to do something that was suggested to us. How can we do this?

We were all made in God's image, and we have to remind ourselves of this, because if we are saying these things about ourselves, we are also saying them about God. We are all God's children, and we are all wonderfully made. We may be different in looks, or knowledge, or in our relationship with Christ, but we are all perfect in his sight, and so we need to not tear ourselves down.

How sad God must be when we talk down about ourselves. Did we ever make something that we thought was wonderful and was told that it wasn't? Didn't it just break our heart? We need to use that tongue to tell ourselves every morning that we are the child of God, and we are wonderfully made and God loves us.

❧ John 3:16

"For God so loved the world, that he gave his only begotten son, so that anyone who believes in him shall not perish, but have everlasting life."

17.
Protection

Have we ever known anyone that had a rock collection before? These rock collectors will hunt for different rocks, and then take them home and label them. They will spend hours examining them, and turning them around at different angles to try to see what the rock is composed of, and what different minerals run through the core of it. They are probably the same people who love to go through the caverns, and see the stalagmites, and the stalactites. They can explain to the person next to them how these rock formations were formed, they are just a wealth of knowledge when it comes to what we would consider just a plain old rock.

What is it about rocks that fascinate people? Little boys are notorious for picking up rocks, and carrying them in their pockets. I've seen "pet rocks" in stores, and I have even seen "worry stones" for people to carry with them, to rub their fingers on when they become stressed or anxious.

I will even admit to having a rock, not a whole rock collection, but just one rock that I keep. My mother in law introduced me to a friend of hers from Nova Scotia, and this woman had a collection of river rocks that she had brought with her from Nova Scotia. This woman was kind enough to offer me one of these rocks, as I had never seen one before. It looks like just a plain ordinary rock, small enough to hold in the palm of my hand, and it has a smooth surface. Now, run this same rock under a stream of water, and it becomes beautiful, with different shades of greens, and spots that appear on it. When I let it dry, it looks like just a plain old rock again.

There's another rock though that we all should have. One that is a MUST have for our collection. It is definitely better than the sand, and mineral combination rocks that we normally find. It is Jesus Christ, our Rock, and our Salvation. He is the rock that we need to build the foundation of our lives on. He is the only solid, reliable, unchanging thing about this life that we live in. He is the same today as he was yesterday, and the same as he will be tomorrow.

We can go to him when we are sad, or sick, or hurt, and we will always find him strong, solid, and unshakable, just like a rock wall. We can go to him, and hide ourselves in this stone fortress. "Rock of Ages cleft for me, let me hide myself in thee." He will make an opening for us to hide in, and find rest, while he guards us from the dangers of this life.

We should take lessons from the natural instinct that the animals have. When an animal is sick or injured, it will go off by itself and hide, to either heal or die, whichever the case might be. We hear of them wondering onto higher ground away from the others, and they will usually seek out a cave, or a ledge in which to be alone; just it and the rock, alone to face whatever comes next.

Birds also, such as the eagle, will build their nests up high on a rocky ledge, because they know that this offers the best protection from the elements, predators and the storms of life. If an eagle becomes ill, it is said that it will fly up to the highest point of the mountain, and find a smooth ledge in which to lie face down on the rock, and stretch its' wings out. It will stay in this position, and let the sun and the heat of the rock, draw the poisons from its system.

When was the last time we were sick or ill, either emotionally, or physically, or both? Did we partake of something that was bad for us? Maybe some form of sin that made us so ill, we actually felt like we were dying? Maybe we were even wishing that we would, just to put us out of our misery!

Did we head straight for the only one that could help us? Did we crawl away to higher ground and seek a smooth rock upon which we could lay, while we let the "Son" draw the poison out of us? Did we search for a cave, or a crevice in the "Rock?" Were we alone, just us and the shelter of the Rock, until we were strong enough again to continue on our journey?

Next time we are hurting, let's not wait; we need to run, not walk to higher ground. Just like the Rocky Mountains, Jesus will always be there to offer us his shelter, his strength, and his protection.

Why don't we go ahead and crawl up on that "Rock", and stretch out our wings, and find rest for our weary self, and let the "Son" warm us with the heat of his love.

✒ Psalms 18:2-3

"The Lord is my fort where I can enter and be safe; no one can follow me in and slay me. He is a rugged mountain where I hide; he is my Savior, a rock where none can reach me, and a tower of safety. He is my shield."

18.
Satisfaction

How many of us spend hours daydreaming of what we could have been, or what we could have done, if only we would have had the chance. Do we realize how much time we have truly wasted in this past time?

We say things like these on a regular basis. "If only my parents had been rich." "If only I had been an only child." "If only I had graduated high school." "If only I had gone to college." "If only I was married, or not married." "If only I had kids, or didn't have kids." The list is endless, with literally hundreds of possible scenarios.

Are we ever going to be able to be satisfied with where we are? Can we be satisfied with the spouse, and kids God gave us? With the job, and home that God has provided?

Have we ever agonized over something that we thought we really wanted or felt we needed to have? Have we pleaded with God to give it to us, and rationalized it to everyone around us? Have we even told ourselves that if we could just have that one thing, we wouldn't need, or want anything else?

Now, I'm sure that it has not happened all the time, but there have probably been times when we have gotten "our heart's desire." Now what? Are we happy? Have we never asked for another thing since?

No. Why? Because, that is our human nature to always want more; the bigger house, that becomes a chore to clean; the sports car that looks good until the next year's model comes out; the dream job with the hidden quirks that we weren't aware of.

Today's economy has been a big wake up call for so many people. Sadly, it has not necessarily been a pleasant wake up call. So many people that have been living beyond their financial limit now find themselves unemployed, and their homes in foreclosure. Other people find themselves with huge mounds of credit card debt. Why? Because everyone is trying to fill a void in our lives with things, like the bigger house, the higher paying job, and the sports car.

We need to learn to enjoy where we are at the moment. We miss so much of the present because we are striving for tomorrow. But you know what? Tomorrow never comes, nor is tomorrow promised to any of us. We are not to build up our riches here on earth.

If we have food, shelter, our health, family, and work, then we have enough. We have to tell ourselves that we have enough and be satisfied.

Ecclesiastes 6:19-20, "It is very good if a man has received wealth from the Lord, and the good health to enjoy it. To enjoy your work and to accept your lot in life, that is indeed a gift from God. The person who does that will not need to look back with sorrow on his past, for God gives him joy."

How many people are missing out on enjoying the present, and missing out on their children growing up because they feel they have to work long hours. Now, I understand that there are people who are seriously in financial straits, and must work more just to survive, but I'm talking about the ones who are doing it because they want more. Yeah, our kids enjoy the vacations, and the latest video games, but I bet they would enjoy spending time at home with us just as much. Kids need and want their parents love and attention, and we can't be properly giving it to them if we're out chasing the American dream, or the mighty dollar.

We need to accept our life, and live each day to the fullest. If we are blessed to have more, wonderful, enjoy it, maybe even bless someone else with some of it. If we aren't, accept it according to God's word, and enjoy what we've been given so far.

If we really think we need something, we should take it to the Lord in prayer. If we still don't get it, we should assume that for some reason God feels we don't need it at this time. Sometimes, if we can learn to be content without it, God will bless us with something even better later on.

Find contentment in today. Sometimes, it's the little things that add up to the biggest blessings in our lives, like the little things that we originally overlooked in our pursuit of the bigger and better. We need to stop, and stand still for just a minute and look around us and say "this is the day the Lord hath made, I will rejoice and be glad in it!"

❧ Hebrews 13:9

"Stay away from the love of money; be satisfied with what you have. For God has said, "I will never, never fail you nor forsake you."

19.
Size

Does size really matter? We have heard that phrase used in many different contexts, and relating to many different things. Does size matter? I guess it depends on the conversation. When I hear that phrase, something different comes to my mind.

Does size matter when we are purchasing a cheeseburger? Sure. We don't want to spend the money thinking we getting a whopper and we are given a child's size burger.

Does size matter when purchasing a house? Sure. We don't want to purchase a small home when we have six kids.

Does size matter when we are looking at other people? Sure it does, if we are truly looking at the other person.

Maybe that is a little odd, but it's true, the size of a person does matter; but only the size of that person's heart. Not their dress size, their weight, or how tall they are.

I was raised in a large family, with three girls, and three boys. I was the middle girl. We were also a large family in body size, especially the girls.

I was raised in the 70's, when all the models where thin, and like many women, I have had body issues all my life, but as I have aged, I realize the perfect body does not exist.

I know there are health risks associated with obesity, like high blood pressure, diabetes, and high cholesterol. I am dealing with some of these issues myself.

But as I grow older, I feel that some things are much more important than trying to have the perfect body.

A lot of people will say that health is important, and I agree; but the condition of our heart is much more important. When I say that, I do not mean whether our hearts are beating too fast, too slow, or skipping beats, I mean is our heart right with God.

God sees the condition of our heart. God knows if we have opened our heart to him, and to the people around us. God knows if we have shown compassion for our church, and our neighbors.

When we extend a helping hand to another person, are we doing it because of our love for God, or are we doing it to boost our self-esteem. Do we say "Hey look at me!", "Look what I did." Maybe, we are even hoping to be reimbursed in some way.

We have to get our hearts right with God. We have to be spending time in his word, spending time in prayer, and helping our neighbor. This is the kind of activity that God wants to use to get us into shape.

When we meet a person on the street, what is the first thing we notice about them, their eyes, the color of their hair, or maybe their physical features?

BE HONEST! Do we walk away and say to ourselves, "my, she was a big girl", or do we look past the physical features, and walk away thinking "she seemed so nice, I hope I meet up with her again?"

And have we ever seen two people together, and think, "Man, he could have done better than her", or "What do you think she sees in him?" These people have probably looked past the physical features and looked at the heart of the other person.

I have never won any beauty contests myself, and I have done the same thing in the past, I have looked at a person without looking at their heart.

I have met a lot of so called "ugly" people, who had a heart of gold, and would give someone the shirt off their back if need be; but I have also met some beautiful people, with great bodies, beautiful faces, and a mean and nasty heart that was as black as coal.

How do we know who's got a right heart and who doesn't? We don't, unless we get close enough to that person to get to know them. God knows them, he knows who has a right heart, and he will bring these people into our life when we need help, or to help change our heart. Are we going to recognize them, or are we going to detour around them because of their looks, like the rest of society?

LOOK AT THE HEART! REMEMBER GOD SEES OUR HEART!

I've been questioned before about my diet plan, or my eating program, and inquiries regarding how am I going to get my body back in shape, because once again I've gained all my weight back after losing it. But you know what? It's not about diet plans, and eating programs, or which gym to go to. It's not!

This body we have, is only temporary, we're not keeping it forever. This is only a shell. We will have new bodies in heaven, but first we have to get there, and we'll only get there through Christ Jesus. We have to accept Jesus as our savior, and invite him into our hearts.

Believe me, our bodies might be big, but our hearts are bigger, big enough to allow Jesus to live in, and big enough to hold love for our friends and family.

When God looks at us, he sees our heart, not our body. Why don't we start today to do the same, and stop being so concerned with our dress size, and start to be concerned with the size of our heart? Instead of working on the outside, let's work on the inside, after all, beauty is only skin deep.

Next time we see that other person, look at their heart.

Now, does size matter? Go ahead and skip the double cheeseburger if you want, but don't skip out on the double portion of God's love and grace, that he has for those who love and honor him.

❧ 1 Peter 3:3-4

"Don't be concerned about the outward beauty. Be beautiful inside, in your hearts, with the lasting charm of a gentle and quiet spirit which is so precious to God."

20.
Grace

Have we ever felt like we were totally drained? I mean just drained mentally, emotionally, and physically. Not from a recent bout with the flu or a stomach bug. I mean from your dealings with other people.

I know there are a lot of store clerks or healthcare workers out there that will say "yeah, that's me every day!" Any type of job, that deals with the public, day in and day out, can be exhausting.

We have to smile and be pleasant while the other person can be "chewing our head off", for every wrong they feel that we personally committed against them. Now sure, we're compensated for this grief with a paycheck every week, and hopefully, most weeks it works out even.

What about the people that we don't get paid to be nice to, like maybe a relative, or a coworker. Maybe it's a friend that we've known since high school. Whoever it is, they are the ones that completely drain our energy. They are the ones that can exhaust us until there is literally nothing left for anyone else.

We've probably all known someone like that, haven't we? She's the one that clings to us constantly; dropping by our desk every half hour to chat. Keeping us from our necessary tasks, and then she walks off in a huff, if we are too busy at the moment to talk. The one that is now mad at us, because she is so insecure that she feels we slighted her, and thinks we no longer want to be her friend. Even though we had already spoken to her the last five times she stopped by.

Maybe it's the relative that we really love, but dread calling. We can't get a word in edge wise, as they tell us all about the latest ills, and health issues, they imagine they have.

Maybe it's the friend who has lived through a tragedy in the past, like a spouse that had left them. Even though it happened years ago, this is still the current topic of conversation every time we get together.

There are a lot of "walking wounded" that are searching for other people to be their crutch. They feel that they just can't make it on their own without someone else to lean on.

Now, as Christians, we are called to serve others, and to show God's love to others through our deeds, but we need to use caution.

Maybe we started out by showing someone kindness, or helping them to get through some tragedy that fell upon them. But this should only have been for the short term, until they were strong enough to stand on their own two feet again. But that's the problem, because some of them are never able to stand alone. Maybe this is something new, or maybe they have always been like this.

The problem, just like quicksand, is that we don't notice it until we're stuck in it and can't get out! Now, we're knee deep and they're trying to pull us in deeper. We can't help anyone else because we're stuck, and we're exhausted from struggling against it and getting nowhere.

There's only one thing to do. We have to get out and seek higher ground. Seek Jesus to help pull us out of the mire and set our feet back on solid ground. Then we need to slowly start distancing ourselves from that quicksand pit.

You see, what will happen is, if we don't get ourselves out, we will be stuck there with the other person pulling us down until we both drown in it. Then we've lost our ability to help anyone else because we couldn't, or wouldn't leave that pit.

Please don't stay in the quicksand out of a sense of loyalty to the other person. Most of these people prefer to stay there, even after we've offered them the assistance to get out. And don't worry, because someone else will be along shortly to try to talk them out of it just like we did.

Now, when I say distance ourselves, sometimes that's just not possible. Maybe the person is a close relative or a coworker that we see every day. There is just no way to avoid them.

We need to pray about it and try to limit our exposure to them. Maybe cut back on the length of time we spend on the phone with "Aunt Mildred." Give her a quick call every day, but limit it to no more than ten minutes. If it is a coworker, explain that we can't chat all the time, or have lunch together every day. Limit it to maybe a cup of coffee at break time for five minutes, or maybe lunch only once a week.

Continue to cover them in prayer, and hopefully they won't always need a human crutch. Hopefully, they will find Jesus to lean on.

❧ Psalms 10:17-18

"Lord, you know the hope of humble people. Surely you will hear their cries and comfort their hearts by helping them. You will be with the orphans and all who are oppressed, so that mere earthly man will terrify them no longer."

21.
Words

How many times have we walked along a gravel road and gotten a rock in our shoe? That really hurts, doesn't it? It hurts bad enough that most people I know will stop immediately, and take their shoe off to get the pebble out. Even after the pebble is out, and we continue to walk, the spot on our foot is still bruised and tender, sometimes for a few days afterward.

Have we ever imagined being hit with a rock, maybe in the chest or the face, and feeling the pain from the stone's impact, and the feeling of blood starting to trickle? Can we imagine being struck by the rocks, over and over again, from all directions, and being unable to stop them? Rocks that were thrown by friends, neighbors, even some family members, and meant to kill us.

This was the fate of the woman who committed adultery as recorded in John Chapter 8. She was brought before a crowd of people, as well as Jesus, and sentenced to death by having stones thrown at her until she died. What a horrible fate!

Would we want that kind of punishment inflicted on people found guilty in our day and age? Could we watch people become cut, bruised, and bloody? Well, guess what? It is happening, right here, all around us. We don't see it? Well trust me, it's happening, and we've probably thrown a few of those stones ourselves.

You see, the stones are really not stones, but words, and I believe they can cut, and bruise just the same.

We know the hectic life we are all living, taking care of the house, the job, and the kids; we are stretched like a rubber band, and all it takes is one more thing, added by some poor unsuspecting person, to make us snap. Then the rock is in the slingshot, and we've aimed, and fired before we gave our mind a chance to stop our mouth.

Maybe it was the cashier at the supermarket, who we felt was moving too slow; maybe it's a co-worker, who asked us to help them with something, when we really couldn't spare the time; or maybe it's our spouse that we hurl rocks at as soon as they come in the door.

It doesn't matter who it is, but if they get in our way we will stone them. To death if need be.

Now the stones serve their purpose, one smart remark, or curse word spoken, and that other person will think twice before bothering us again, but is this what we really want? Is this how we really want to be perceived?

Sometimes, we've been on the receiving end of a stoning, haven't we? Just out of the blue, someone snaps at us with a harsh, or unkind word, or some smart remark to make us feel stupid, and like with the slingshot, the hit is taken before we know it is coming. Now, we walk away with a cut, or a bruise, and sometimes, if we were particularly close to that person, the cut is deeper, and the pain more intense, and the tender, sore spot lasts a whole lot longer. Even after apologies are made, the spot can stay tender and sometimes never completely heal.

Why do we do this to each other? If we're the one that hurled the stone, we may actually feel better for a moment, and then the guilt sets in. The Holy Spirit will nudge us and ask "What just happened here?", but we have no answer for it, because most of the time, we don't know what happened. We just snapped!

What we need is more prayer time. I know we have no room to squeeze it in, right?

Well, if our mornings are busy, trying to get everyone out the door, how about a five minute conversation with God while we're driving to work, or maybe each time we use the restroom. We can give him thanks for getting us through the morning as we're waiting for the microwave to heat our lunch. Maybe, we could ask him to be with us again tomorrow as we're setting the table for supper.

Remember, God wants to be there for us, and just like any parent, he doesn't like to see his children hurting each other.

Talking things over with God as they happen throughout the day can be a big stress reliever. The conversations don't have to be long, maybe just a few words, or a sentence or two each time.

We all know what it feels like to be hit with a rock, it hurts, so let's put our slingshots away.

❧ James 1:26

"Anyone who says he is a Christian but doesn't control his sharp tongue is just fooling himself, and his religion isn't worth much."

22.
Stumbling Block

We never know what God might use in order to speak to someone, so we need to be very careful that we don't inject ourselves between God and someone as a stumbling block.

Usually, we do this by imposing our own opinions, or our beliefs, on to that person, which will cause them to lose ground in their walk with God. We are all different human beings, in our ideas, our opinions, even in our backgrounds, such as how we were raised. Unless, we are directly from the same family, we just don't know what the other person is feeling, or thinking in different situations; we can only know what we are thinking or feeling.

Now, everyone's relationship with God is just as different. What we talk to God about, and what he tells one person to do or not do, may seem very strange if we knew, and vice versa; so, in saying that, we need to be very careful to keep from telling other people what their next step should be, unless, of course, we are praying together as a group, for specific directions on something.

For instance, people have specific ideas as to what other people should wear to church. Some churches prefer women to wear only dresses, and the men to wear suits and ties. Other churches are more relaxed, and liberal with their dress code. Either way, we want to make sure that we are not giving a visitor to our church, a look, or a comment, that says they are not dressed well enough to attend our church, or that they won't fit in.

How many of us have ever attended a function, only to discover that we were not dressed properly for the occasion? It's awkward, isn't it, and we feel that we stick out like a sore thumb. Now, add a few sly looks from other people, or a whispered comment from one person to another, and we're anxious to leave, and usually vow to never return.

Do we imagine that God approves of this? I've wondered before, how far back through the ages, that it became necessary to wear only our "best" to church.

God did not say that we can only gather to worship if we are "dressed to the nines." Christ said "Where two or more are gathered in my name, I will be present." He didn't say how we had to be dressed.

Many people feel that they can't attend church services because they don't have the proper clothes, or they are too uncomfortable being dressed up; but they have a desire to seek God, so maybe, they show up at church, in a pair of jeans and sneakers, and sit uncomfortably through the service, because they are aware of the stares they receive. Do we think they will want to come back next Sunday? Would we, if the tables were turned?

WWJD? What would Jesus do? Would he prefer that this person come, just as they are, and hear a message about God's love and forgiveness, or would he prefer that this person sit at home, and miss this opportunity to hear God's word, because they were wearing a pair of jeans and a T-shirt? Is this what God is really about?

Never! Jesus is about spreading the Good News of his salvation to everyone, not just to the ones who are dressed up, and come to church every Sunday.

Do we think that the missionaries are dressing up the natives before they give them the gospel message? Hardly!

Also, when we encourage others to read the Bible, are we right to say absolutely that one particular Bible translation is correct, and all the others are wrong? If that's the case, a lot of the Bible translators, who have spent their whole lives translating the Bible into other languages have just wasted all of their work, after all, the words may not be exactly the same as the King James Version once it is in another language.

Now again, WWJD? Should we continue to tell people to read no other translation of the Bible? Should we tell people that they can't read a different translation of the Bible, even though it may be easier for them to follow and understand? After all, we want people to learn about Jesus, but if they can't understand what they're reading, it won't do them any good; or they will not bother to even read it at all, and Jesus wants us to be in his word.

Let's keep these things in mind when we are talking with other people. Jesus can use anything he chooses to tell his story. Please don't be a stumbling block to stop others from getting to know, and hear God's messages.

❧ 1 Corinthians 3:11

"And no one can ever lay any other real foundation than that one we already have-Jesus Christ. But there are various kinds of materials that can be used to build on that foundation."

23.
Sickness

I have heard people say, "I've never been sick a day in my life." Do they really mean that? I think that what they really mean is that they don't have a chronic illness, or a major health crisis, that they have dealt with. But really, can any of us say that we have never been sick a day in our life? No, because sickness comes to all of us, and it comes to our families, our neighbors, and our friends also. It's not picky who it lands on, and tries to devour.

We may not all deal with the same health issues, but we will all get our turn at dealing with something, it's inevitable. And just like the rain that falls from the sky, sickness, disease, and death, will fall on the just, and the unjust people alike.

Many people question God's motives when one of his people fall prey to illness. They rant, and rave, at God for not being there for them, or their loved one. They say "God, they were a Christian, why them?" and, "Where were you God when we needed you?" If you believe anything at all, believe me when I say God was there, and is still there, and he has not left us alone, not for one second.

God is in control of our situation. We know that he can heal the sick, and raise the dead, but we have to remember that if he does, hallelujah; but if he doesn't, then that was God's will, and we have to know that it somehow fits into his plan for us.

And just like when Lazarus died, Jesus weeps with us. John 11:35 tells us "Jesus wept." When was the last time we wept because of a health issue that had us scared, and uncertain? Maybe it was a condition that had us in pain, or even disabled. How about a cancer diagnosis for our self, or a loved one, or a doctor telling us that they've tried all they know to do? How many of us have been there? Maybe we're there now, if we're not, we will be sometime during this lifetime.

But the good news is that God is with us, and he's there to comfort us, to strengthen us, to weep with us, and to dry our tears. We just need to turn, and fall into his arms because he's waiting to give us all we need.

In John 11:25, Jesus said "I am the one who raises the dead and gives them life again. Anyone who believes in me, even though he dies, he shall live again. He will be given eternal life and shall never perish." Our time here on earth will last only for a moment, but our time in heaven is for an eternity! Romans 8:18, "What we suffer now is nothing compared to the glory He will give us later. No more sickness. No more pain."

Jesus became flesh, and came to earth, but he also was not exempt from suffering. Can we just picture ourselves walking for miles at a time in the hot, dry, and dusty country, wouldn't our legs, and feet hurt? After we have walked for hours in the sun, wouldn't our skin get sun burnt and our throat be parched? If we were sleeping on the ground, wouldn't our bodies be stiff and achy? Then, what if we're beaten, and nailed to a cross to die? Yes, I believe he also knew suffering.

What I'm going to say next is probably going to sound strange, but I feel God is leading me to say this. When we ourselves are suffering, or if we are standing by while a loved one is suffering, we still need to give praise to God. Praise God from where-ever we are. If we can't go to him, ask and he will make himself known to us, because he is already with us.

If our legs are weak or crippled, and we can't kneel to pray, or stand up in church, or even walk to the altar, we can praise him from our seat in the pew, or our wheelchair. If we are suffering from a heart or lung issue, and we can't sing out loud, we can sing his praises silently to our self. If we are home bound and can't attend church, God will meet us in our own living room or bedroom.

If we feel that we can't quite bring ourselves to praise him through our illness or trial, then we can offer him what we are able to give; and thank him for whatever we can. Maybe thank him that we don't have a headache today, thank him that we were able to get out of bed, or that we were able to walk into the bathroom, whatever it might be. Remember that the Holy Spirit is in us, and he prays for us when we are not even sure what we should be praying for, or how we should pray. So if we are too sick to offer up our own prayers or praise, we can just sit quietly and let the Holy Spirit help us; that's why he was given to us.

Romans 8:36-39 "We must be ready to face death at every moment of the day for we don't know when it will be. But what we do know is that Christ died for us because he loves us and no matter what we are going through during our time on this earth, there is NOTHING that can ever separate us from his love. Death can't, and life can't. The angels in heaven won't and all the powers of hell cannot keep God's love away from us.

So let's fall into his arms, and receive his love and comfort, because when we are hurting the worst, that's when he wants to love, and comfort us the most!

❧ Romans 8:23

"And even we Christians, although we have the Holy Spirit within us as a foretaste of future glory, also groan to be released from pain and suffering. We, too, wait anxiously for that day when God will give us our full rights as his children, including the new bodies he has promised us-bodies that will never be sick again and will never die."

24.
Temptations

The devil made me do it! How many times have we heard that excuse? Well, it's true, temptations are all around us. James 1:14 tells us that a temptation is the pull of man's own evil thoughts and wishes. These evil thoughts then lead to evil actions, but what we need to remember is that James also tells us in 1:13, these temptations do not come from God. We should remember that a temptation is an evil thought that leads to an evil action, and God is NEVER associated with evil.

The devil will plant different seeds, or ideas, into our thoughts to see what we will finally act on. Now the devil usually already knows what will work for each of us, depending on our family history. You see, if our ancestors had trouble with alcohol or drugs, chances are we will be more susceptible to this temptation. That's why it seems like these things are passed from parent to child, or that certain wrong behaviors, such as sexual sins, or abuse tend to "run in families."

When we actually allow ourselves to act on a temptation is when we sin. We all fall to one temptation or another, it's unavoidable. You see, if we strengthen our resolve to push the devil back in one area of temptation, he will just return with something different, and then later with something else. He will keep trying until he finds the right "lure." Just like with a fishing tackle box, the devil has different lures for different people, the same as a fisherman has different lures for different fish. What might easily tempt one person might not tempt another person at all, and vice versa.

Nobody is exempt from temptations, not even Jesus. We know from the scriptures that Jesus was led into the wilderness and tempted in every way. We need to remember this, he was tempted in every way, so it doesn't matter what the temptation is, Jesus has already faced it, and conquered it.

We have to be watchful, and on alert all the time against these attacks of temptation. Some of the time they can be small, like disobeying the speed limit, or bigger ones like adultery, or huge ones like murder.

Sometimes the devil will even use other people in our lives to tempt us into doing wrong. Have we ever had someone make a suggestion to do something that we knew was wrong, but they just kept chipping away at our resolve? It usually starts out with a suggestion, and then they will coax us, sometimes they even become angry at us, until we finally give in just to get them off our back. Jesus said in Luke 17:1-2 "There will always be temptations to sin, but woe to the man who does the tempting." He goes on to say "It would be better for the person doing the tempting to have a huge rock tied around their neck and thrown into the sea." Wow, that is scary.

This passage leads me to believe that we must be very cautious not to tempt others to sin, so if there is something in our lives that we are doing wrong, we need to make sure we are not tempting others to follow us.

We can also be tempted by things we see or hear, such as reading, or watching porn, can tempt people to commit sexual sins, such as adultery, rape or incest.

We sometimes put ourselves in a position to listen to gossip or profanity; or we watch movies that tempt us to commit violent or destructive acts towards property, or other people.

We need to pray about our temptations, and bring our weakness before God so that he can strengthen us to resist. He will always provide us with a way out of a temptation, most of the time, it is as simple as giving us the strength to just say "No!"

We need to also learn other behaviors that will assist us, when possible, to resist temptation. For example, if we know there is always a lot of gossip in the break room, try finding another spot to eat our lunch so that we avoid joining in on such conversations.

Block the cable TV channels, or remove the internet if this is a temptation for us to watch porn, or violent movies.

Mostly, just remember that whatever the temptation is, we need to bring it to God. We also need to stay close to him so that he can protect us, and give us strength when we feel weak, and ready to give in to the temptations of this life.

❧ James 1:12

"Happy is the man who doesn't give in and do wrong when he is tempted, for afterwards he will get as his reward the crown of life that God has promised to those who love him."

25.
Tithes

God has said "I will open up the windows of heaven for you, and pour out a blessing so great, you won't have room enough to take it in" Wow! I don't know what everyone else thinks about that, but it gets me excited! A blessing so big there's no room for it, because it's bigger than a house, even if we rented a conference center, or a stadium, God says we still wouldn't have room for it. Can we even imagine something being that huge; a blessing that is so big, nothing on earth could contain it? Now, I know we're all running to the front of the line to get in on that, right? Sign me up too! We just have to do one little thing first. Are you ready to hear what it is? I'll just warn you, it might be difficult.

We have to tithe. "Bring all the tithes into the storehouse so there will be food enough in my temple. If you do, I will open the windows of heaven and pour out a blessing." This is the instruction God has given in Malachi 3:10.

I said it may be difficult. People get defensive when we are told what we should do with our belongings, especially our money. But, what we don't understand is, that it's not our money, it's God's money.

He has given it to us to manage, and he expects us to do good things with it. All he asks is that we give him back his portion that is owed to him.

We need to be like the poor widow woman in Luke 21:1-3, she gave her last two pennies, while the rich man did not give enough money for him to even notice the loss from his bank account.

Are we able to gladly give our last two pennies to God, or to anyone?

I have seen many people who have come to church for the message, but when the offering plate is passed they put nothing in it. Nothing! I have heard people say "I just don't have it", or "I'm short on funds this week." Like the widow woman, we are told to give regardless. She didn't have it to give. She was short on funds. That was her last two pennies!

Have we ever gotten down to our last two pennies? If we did, I bet we were holding on tight to them. After all, that's all we had, right?

God says we are to give generously and with a joyous heart. Matthew 6:25 tells us, we are not to worry about "things", like food, clothes, and drink. God will provide. It doesn't specify, but money is considered a "thing."

We are not to store up treasures here on earth, and to give with a joyous heart. The bible says it is harder for a rich man to get into heaven, than for a camel to pass through the eye of a needle. Why is that?

Maybe it is because money is the bargaining tool of the age. We can buy anything with it, all the fancy clothes, the cars, and the big houses; the funny thing is, the more we have, the more we want, so then the more money we need. Money is power, and it can sometimes get out of control!

We are told to live simply. If God has blessed us well financially, than we are to pass that on to help others. We are also told to return to God his portion of everything given to us.

Why? He is God, what would he need with money? This is not about God needing money. Hello! He's God! It's about our obedience to him and to his word. If we can be obedient in the smaller things, God will bless us with bigger things.

"Bring all the tithes to the storehouse so there will be food enough in my temple." The church is the storehouse, and we are to bring our tithes to God at his place of worship.

I hear people also complain that "the church doesn't need money", or that "the preacher doesn't need money." They say "I have a wealthy church." We are told to take care of our preachers, so that they can minister to God's flock (his people). If there is a preacher who is abusing the church funds, he will answer to God directly, for the bible tells us that preachers, and teachers of the gospel, are held at a much higher standard. If they have caused someone to stop believing as a result of their actions, I really would not want to be in their shoes on Judgment Day!

"So there will be food enough in my temple." The churches are to use the tithes to pass on the gospel to those who have not heard it. Remember, Jesus is called the Bread of Life. There needs to be enough financial resources, to assist the missionaries throughout the world, to pass this message of Jesus on to others, and when they do this, they are feeding the masses.

Remember to give God his portion so that we can be richly blessed and prove our obedience.

Doesn't it feel good knowing that we also are helping to "feed the hungry?"

Proverbs 3:9-10

"Honor the Lord by giving him the first part of all your income, and he will fill your barns with wheat and barley, and overflow your wine vats with the finest wines."

26.
Waiting

Have we ever thought about how much people can resemble birds? Not just in looks, although I have seen people with features that resemble birds, such a person with a hook nose like a hawk, or legs like a chicken.

But I'm talking more about their actions. Haven't we heard expressions before, like people getting their feathers ruffled, or acting like a mother hen, or maybe our grandchildren chatting like a magpie; maybe someone else getting mad as an old wet hen, strutting around like a rooster, or being proud as a peacock?

Isn't it funny how we compare people to birds? Well, did we know that the bible also has references regarding birds? Not the magpies, or roosters, or peacocks (even though a lot of the Pharisees could have resembled the peacocks). The bible refers to eagles.

Exodus 19:4

"Ye have seen what I did unto the Egyptians and how I bare you on eagles' wings and bring you unto myself".

Deuteronomy 28:49

"The Lord shall be as swift as the eagle flieth."

Job 39:27

"Though thou exalt thyself as the eagle and set thy nest among the stars…thence will I bring thee down, saith the Lord."

Hosea 8:1

"He shall come as an eagle against the house of the Lord."

But my favorite verse in the bible is **Isaiah 40:31**

"But they that wait upon the Lord shall renew their strength; they shall mount up with wings as eagles; they shall run and not be weary; and they shall walk and not faint."

That verse is so refreshing, and so inspiring. When we've run ourselves ragged, with the jobs, and the house, and the kids or grandkids, and the everyday mundane things, that make us tired and worn out, we can go to the Lord, and he will renew our strength! They (us) shall run and not be weary. I don't know about you, but some days, I'm just weary getting out of bed, and thinking of everything that needs to be done, but the Lord will RENEW MY STRENGTH!

Let me say that again. When we wait upon the Lord, he will renew our strength. But do we wait upon the Lord? Do we sit back and say, "Ok Lord, here's the problem, you deal with it?" NO! We run to our families, our friends, maybe even to our coworkers for advice regarding the problem first. Then we might talk to our spouse and get their opinion; informing our spouse of everyone else's opinions, and together try to decide how to deal with it. We might throw up a half-hearted "help me Lord", but do we honestly ask for his help first? Do we honestly sit back and wait for him to take care of things?

Don't we sometimes wonder what God sees when he looks down at us? He's expecting us to give him our burdens and problems, and for us to wait on him for our answers. But what he sees probably resembles us as a mouse, and the solution to our problem is the cheese at the end of the maze. Can we picture it? We are running helter-skelter through this maze, running into dead ends, and road blocks, back tracking, and trying to look over the sides of the maze. We know we can get to the end, if we just keep running around fast enough, or long enough. Now we are more like a chicken with its head cut off.

And why are we running around like a chicken with our head cut off? We will eventually get the solution to our problem, but in God's own way, and in his own timing. That is when we will get it. So we don't need to be running around, and wearing ourselves out.

If we would just learn to wait upon the Lord, the Lord will renew our strength. We shall run and not be weary, we shall walk and not faint, and we shall mount up with wings as eagles.

I heard a story once about a farmer who had found a baby eagle, and he clipped its wings, and kept it in the chicken coop with his chickens. The story told how different the eagle was compared to the chickens. The eagle didn't gather into a huddle with the other chickens when they heard a noise, or squawk endlessly all day.

No, that eagle was very different. He kept to himself and was more subdued than the chickens. He didn't run at every noise. He stood his ground, and you know what else he did? He watched the sky; he was always looking up and scanning the horizon. He would stand for hours just watching the sky.

Then the story went on to say how the farmer had neglected to continue to clip the eagles' wings, until one day a storm came; of course the chickens all started to squawk at each other, and run in circles, tripping each other on their way to the coop, where I'm sure they huddled together with their heads tucked under their wings.

But that little eagle didn't run. He welcomed the storm. He even turned with his face into the storm, because he wasn't afraid. When the wind blew harder, he stretched out his wings and let the wind ruffle through his feathers.

Do we welcome the storms, and stretch out our arms when the storms of life come along and ruffle our feathers? Or do we run together, squawking and hiding in our coop with our heads covered?

Next, that eagle jumped up on a post and stood with his wings out, and he gave his wings a few trial flaps; as the thunder was rolling, and the lightning was flashing all around, that eagle stood with his wings outstretched and caught the wind current, and he was off! He was flying higher, and higher, circling the chicken coop where he had been, flying higher and closer to the heavens. He didn't care about the storm. He embraced it! He knew he wasn't a chicken like the others, and he didn't want to stay on the ground, and peck the dirt, and run at every noise. He wasn't a chicken, he was an eagle, and he was just waiting to grow and get stronger. He was WAITING to be delivered from his problem. In this case, it was his captivity.

What problem are we in the midst of? What are we being held captive by? Did the devil clip our wings? Are we watching the skies for an answer to our difficulties, or are we running to the coop? Are we standing strong with our wings stretched out to embrace the storm, or are we in a corner with all the other chickens, with our head under our wing?

When we WAIT upon the Lord, he will renew our strength. We will mount up with wings as eagles! Don't be like the mouse in the maze, or the chicken in the coop!

Don't be afraid when the storms of life come, because they will come, just as sure as the sun rises each day, they will come. We should have no fear, regardless of what the storm is in life, whether it is money related, work related, or problems with relationships, such as with friends, family, or coworkers.

The only thing that matters is how we handle the storms when they come. We need to stand firm, always look up and watch the skies, and embrace it. Most of all….Wait on the Lord. Don't tire our self out trying to fix it. We can't! God can, but we can't!

They that wait upon the Lord shall renew their strength. They shall mount up with wings as eagles; they shall run and not be weary; and they shall walk and not faint.

I don't know about you, but I not only want that renewed strength and stamina, but I also want to soar! Just like the eagle, I want to stand, and stretch my wings, and soar into the air, and glide without worrying about the storm around me…God is taking care of the storm!

❧ Psalms 57:1

> "O God, have pity, for I am trusting you! I will hide beneath
> the shadow of your wings until this storm is past."

27.
Whispers

Have we heard from God today? Are we agonizing over something, and we really want an answer from him? How many times have we lain awake at night, worrying about tomorrow, just tossing and turning; maybe we get out of bed and roam around the house.

Doesn't it seem like at night, that's when everything has a tendency to close in on us; the worries of the day, the problems with the kids, the stress of our jobs, or the concerns for our elderly parents? These are the same issues that we dealt with throughout the day, so why are we still awake worrying about them at night? I've heard so many people complain, because they can't shut their mind off from the whirlwind of thoughts that just keep coming, and then they can't sleep.

I think this is one of Satan's favorite games to play with us. He likes to take all of our worries, and magnify them, and add the different "what ifs" to each one. "What if...I tell her this tomorrow" and then "what if...this happens." The possible endings, and scenarios, that we play in our minds are just unbelievable. And after we think we have finally sorted out everything, Satan will throw another idea at us that we hadn't considered. He's an expert at finding them. That's why he's called the tormentor. He loves to harass God's people. And I can picture God, with an image of him sitting on his throne, and he is shaking his head at us for allowing this stuff to continue.

In the darkest part of the night, God is there, waiting to speak with us, and comfort us; waiting to tell us everything will be ok and for us to rest in him. Isn't that what we're all looking for these days, rest, especially after we've played Satan's game all night? We just want to rest, and to be enveloped in the arms of Jesus, and to just lay our weary head on his shoulder and rest.

When we are quiet and restful, this is when we are most able for God to speak to us. It would be much clearer if God would speak to us out of the clouds, in a loud voice, like he did in the Old Testament; then again, with all the cars, radios and TVs making so much noise, maybe he is and we just can't hear him.

The next time the devil starts his "late night talk show" in our mind, we just need to "turn off the TV in our head." We should try to clear our mind, and picture a large sign that says NO! Just picture in our mind, the capital letters N-O! with an exclamation mark after it because we mean business. We are not going to allow Satan to keep tormenting us, and robbing us of our rest and our joy; even if we have to verbally tell Satan it is time for him to leave and let us alone. We can do that, because God gave us the authority, we just don't use it. We need to order Satan, and his buddies, out of our bed room, and out of the house all together. Let them go torment someone else.

Now, in our mind, we can picture Jesus, sitting on the edge of our bed; he's stroking our hair, and whispering words of love and comfort as we doze off. He is reassuring us that he will be with us the next day, and the day after that, in fact, for all of our days.

Now, when God speaks to us, it is usually more of a knowing, that small voice inside us, telling us what we need to know. It's almost like a whisper. Are we quiet enough to hear God whisper? Sometimes, when we're praying or just sitting quietly, God will whisper to us. It might be an answer to something we have been asking about, or some problem that we have been mulling over; then, suddenly deep inside, God will answer, and we'll "know" what we're supposed to do.

Do we feel that we just don't have time to hear from God? Maybe our life is so hectic, we just don't have five minutes to go to the bathroom, let alone visit with God. Then, we need to schedule the time.

We need to plan it into our day somewhere. We all have the new I phone, or a date book, we can pencil God in. Maybe we can start out at least once a week for 15 to 30 minutes, longer and more often of course if we're able. Whatever we are able to do.

Now, we need to keep that appointment, just like if we were meeting with a friend for lunch. We can find a quiet spot on the sofa with the TV off, or a park bench; maybe grab a cup of coffee, and just chat with God. We can just let him know how we are, how the kids are, or what's going on at work. Yes, he already knows, but he wants to hear from us; and just maybe, we will hear from him too.

❧ James 1:5-6, 8

"If you want to know what God wants you to do, ask him, and he will gladly tell you, for he is always ready to give a bountiful supply of wisdom to all who ask him: But when you ask him, be sure that you really expect him to tell you. If you don't ask with faith, don't expect the Lord to give you any solid answer."

28.
Willing Hands

Do we have something that we are really good at, some hidden talent that we have, like singing or writing poetry; maybe we have natural talent for playing a musical instrument. Whatever it is, there is something that each of us enjoy doing.

1 Peter 4:10 tells us that God has given each of us special abilities or talents. Whatever that ability is, we are told to use it. God wants each of us to use our abilities in some form, not only to honor him, but also to further his kingdom.

Maybe we sing, if so, invite some friends to hear us sing at church, either as a solo performance, or in the choir. If we dance or do ballet, ask our church about forming a dance or drama troupe.

If we like to write, we could submit poetry, or articles, for the church newsletter, or maybe write notes of encouragement to the missionaries in the field. I'm sure they would be happy to hear what's going on in our town or church.

Maybe our talent is cooking, or baking, if so, we could offer our services at a church gathering.

Maybe we like to be busy with our hands, and are good at fixing things, we could offer to fix small things, or do landscaping around the church, or for shut-ins. There is always grass to mow in the summer, and snow to shovel in the winter.

Maybe we feel our only talent was in raising our children, if so, we could work in the nursery and give the mothers a well-deserved break to enjoy the service.

Whatever it is, big or small, God can use us; we just have to be willing. We should be willing to do anything from the most insignificant job, all the way up to the most important. The world may say we have to be qualified for different positions here on earth, but when God is our employer, he will equip us, and make us qualified for whatever position he feels is necessary.

So many people have a servant's heart, and feel the nudge of the Holy Spirit to help, but they don't. Why don't they? Because they feel they aren't good enough, or qualified to do the work. Let God decide who's qualified and who's not.

Believe me, if God feels he can use us somewhere, and we give him the okay, he can qualify us, and have us ready in a hurry. But you see, this is the most important part, we have to give him the okay. Our God is a wonderful and amazing God, and he knows what is best for each of us, but he also gives us a choice. It is our choice whether or not we agree to be used in the manner in which God wants to use us.

Don't get me wrong, there are times when he may use us regardless; if his Divine Plan calls for it, he will place us in a position where we need to be, but we won't always be happy about it. Some-times we'll grumble, and moan, and complain, worse than the Israelites did when God was bringing them through the desert, and if we don't soon straighten ourselves up, and give ourselves an attitude adjustment, we just might end up in this position for the next 40 years! God, forbid something like that should happen!

Most of the time, God prefers that we choose to be used by him willingly. He prefers to have us come to him and say, "Here I am Lord, use me!" Then wait patiently for him to do just that.

Don't be afraid because we think God will automatically send us into the mission field in the wilds of Africa, or somewhere. Yes, he needs people there too, but I think he puts a special calling on our hearts for that.

Most importantly, we have to have a longing for Jesus. We have to want to follow his example of a willing servant, the Jesus who was willing to wash the feet of his disciples.

Are we willing to serve others, our church, and anyone else who needs us, with no thought of their ability to repay us? Remember, we don't have to be qualified, we just need to be willing.

Remember, the world says "Happy are those who rise and rule", but Christ says "Happy are those who stoop and serve."

࿇ James 2:17

"So you see, it isn't enough just to have faith, you must also do good to prove that you have it. Faith that doesn't show itself by good works is no faith at all-it is dead and useless."

29.
Worry

Are we a worry wart that is stressed out all the time, worrying about what might happen? Do we watch the news, and then worry about the whole state of affairs that our country is in? Maybe we are watching constantly for the next terrorist attack.

Maybe we're worrying about the kids, and our spouse, wondering if they are happy, and healthy. Maybe we worry about our finances or our job. Would we be the president of the local Worrier's Anonymous if there was one?

Let's face it. Some people are just born worriers. We can reassure them until we're blue in the face, but they can't help it. It's just the way they are.

We all worry about things, don't get me wrong. We worry about the sick child, or the job lay off, or paying the mortgage on time. These are the normal, day to day worries that we all face. It's called life.

God knows what we need and he will provide it for us.

Matthew 6:26-27, "Look at the birds, they don't worry about what to eat. They don't need to sow or reap, or store up food for your Heavenly Father feeds them. And you are far more valuable to him than they are. Will all your worries add a single moment to your life?"

The Bible is telling us that we shouldn't worry about the everyday mundane things, God is in charge and he knows what we need, and he will provide it.

"And why worry about your clothes? Look at the field lilies. They don't worry about theirs. Yet King Solomon in all his glory was not clothed as beautifully as they are. And if God cares so wonderfully for flowers that are here today and gone tomorrow, won't he more surely care for you?"

What a comforting thought. We don't have to worry about everything. God will provide it all. After all, we are more important to him than the birds, or flowers, right? And he takes care of them.

Watch the birds sometime. They don't have a care in the world. They just sit in the trees and sing their song. They're not worrying about what they're going to eat next.

So many of the burdens that we worry about, and carry around, just weigh us down, and they seldom come to pass anyway. We've wasted all this time, worried about something that never happened.

Matthew 6:34 "So don't be anxious about tomorrow. God will take care of your tomorrow. Live one day at a time." Can we learn to do that? The "what if's" that tomorrow might bring will just drive us crazy. We can't change it anyway. God has already planned our tomorrow out for us. He will take care of it, if we will only give it over to him.

"I know the plans I have for you." You see, only God knows what tomorrow will bring. Let God take care of it. He knows what we will need to get through it. "Take my yoke upon you for it is light." Can we allow ourselves to give up our heavy worries for his light one? This just seems too good to be true, doesn't it?

We do, at times, give ourselves and our burdens to God, but then we don't know what to do with ourselves, so we take them back again. Don't play tug of war with Jesus. As soon as he takes them, then we take it back. He doesn't want us to carry these burdens, and these worries of life by our self. They have a tendency to wear us out. After all, we may only be worried a little about something, but eventually the longer we carry that worry or burden, the heavier, and heavier it becomes, until we are bent under the weight of it.

Give those burdens to Jesus in prayer, every day if we have to, so that we don't carry them alone. The Bible tells us to bring everything to God in prayer, and to pray without ceasing.

Philippians 4:6-7, "Don't worry about anything; instead pray about everything. Tell God your needs, and don't forget to thank him when he answers. If you do this, you will experience God's peace, which is more wonderful than the human mind can understand. His peace will keep your thoughts, and your hearts, quiet and at rest as you trust in Christ Jesus."

༒ Colossians 3:2

"Let heaven fill your thoughts; don't spend your
time worrying about things down here."

30.
Joy

Have we ever watched a horror movie on TV, where the people became zombies? The people in the movie are just walking around in a state of total emotional detachment. They have no facial expressions, and no interaction with other people. They just seem to walk around in a trance. One of the most popular zombie movies is called, "The Night of the Living Dead."

Now take a look around us, really look at some of the people that we pass every day, either on the street, at work, and even at the grocery store. Don't they look unemotional, with no real interaction with other people; maybe they even seem emotionally detached. We, as a society, are slowly becoming like the zombies. We are slowly becoming the actual "living dead."

How have we gotten ourselves into such an entranced state? To many people, life has become mundane, and joyless. Almost like a chore. Is this what our society has become?

When we do stop and ask each other how we are, we get the same response, "I'm fine." Or else, we might get the response, "I'm just so busy!" This last response seems to be the more popular of the two. We are all busy. We are just constantly rushing here and there; oftentimes, I think we've moved so fast that we've left ourselves behind! When we finally reach our destination, we no longer have the same person along, who we started with.

And we are sure moving through life too fast to analyze our feelings, or even take time to think about how we feel. That's why we get the same old bland answer, "I'm fine." But we're not fine. If we just take the time to look at the other people's faces, we would recognize this. Do we really look fine? Most of us don't even make eye contact with the other person, so how do we know whether the other person is fine or not. We seem to avoid each other because we're so busy; we don't even have time to visit over a cup of coffee anymore.

One of the biggest complaints that I hear, is that nobody listens anymore. Why don't we listen to each other? Wives complain that their husbands don't listen to what they have to say, and that their kids don't listen to them. People even complain that their doctor doesn't listen to them when they are sick. We're all talking, but nobody is listening. Our lives are so busy that we can't slow down enough to hear what is being said; we're already thinking about what we have to do next on our agenda. And if nobody is really listening to us, then why should we bother to talk to them.

So we shut down emotionally, and we just move about in our own little world, as we become more and more like a zombie. After all, we tried to talk to other people in the beginning, but nobody listened; and if nobody listens to us that must mean that nobody cares about us. Our zombie like state of mind is us burrowing down into ourselves. We are insulating our feelings of insecurity and unworthiness; we feel that if we aren't important enough for other people to really listen to us, than we are not very important. We feel like we're not good enough for people to waste their time on us.

But what we need to remember is this is the society that we are living in. We can't let the stress of this life make us so numb that we can't connect with other people anymore. We have to re-energize ourselves, and start to reconnect with each other. That's what everyone really wants. Everyone has a void that has to be filled. They want to know that someone, somewhere, cares about them. Everyone needs to feel that they are loved, that's what will fill that void. We can't pass on the promise of God's love to others, if we can't reveal our own love to them.

The same thing applies to us. We have to remember that God loves, and cares for each one of us; after all, God loved us enough to send his only son to die for each one of us.

1 Peter 5:5 "Let him have all your worries and cares, for he is always thinking about you and watching everything that concerns you." When we love someone, we are always thinking about them and if something concerns them, then it concerns us. God loves us in this same way. How do I know? The Bible tells me so. Just like in 1 Peter 5:5 above, and in John 3:16 "For God so loved the world that he gave his only begotten Son, so that anyone who believes in him will not perish but have everlasting life."

Now, we need to fill that void with Jesus. We can start by asking him to fill us with his love until it overflows to all those around us. When we are filled with God, we are truly alive. We just have to smile, and we're happier; we even see the world in a whole different light. We actually want to tell other people about Jesus, because we want them to have what we have.

Don't be like a zombie, and sleepwalk through this life. Wake up and spread the Good News of the Gospel.

❧ Psalms 16:9-11

"Heart, body, and soul are filled with joy. For you will not leave me among the dead; you will not allow your beloved one to rot in the grave. You have let me experience the joys of life and the exquisite pleasures of your own eternal presence."

Notes:

Notes:

Notes:

Notes:

Notes:

Notes:

Notes:

CPSIA information can be obtained at www.ICGtesting.com
Printed in the USA
BVOW041520200911

271492BV00001B/44/P